Rich Remedies

7/8

03/01/12

Betsy,
 Thanks for the great X country tour of Beaver Creek / Pine Valley!
           Best Wishes
              Rich
PS - "Everything in moderation. Including moderation!"

Rich Remedies
My Amazing Natural Self Healing Discoveries

Volume 1

Richard Tyson

iUniverse, Inc.
New York Bloomington Shanghai

Rich Remedies
My Amazing Natural Self Healing Discoveries

Copyright © 2008 by Richard Tyson

All rights reserved. No part of this book may be used or reproduced by any means, graphic, electronic, or mechanical, including photocopying, recording, taping or by any information storage retrieval system without the written permission of the publisher except in the case of brief quotations embodied in critical articles and reviews.

iUniverse books may be ordered through booksellers or by contacting:

iUniverse
1663 Liberty Drive
Bloomington, IN 47403
www.iuniverse.com
1-800-Authors (1-800-288-4677)

Because of the dynamic nature of the Internet, any Web addresses or links contained in this book may have changed since publication and may no longer be valid.

The information, ideas, and suggestions in this book are not intended as a substitute for professional medical advice. Before following any suggestions contained in this book, you should consult your personal physician. Neither the author nor the publisher shall be liable or responsible for any loss or damage allegedly arising as a consequence of your use or application of any information or suggestions in this book.

Book cover art and author photo by Darren Minke. Illustrations and inside photos by Richard Tyson.

ISBN: 978-0-595-49208-4 (pbk)
ISBN: 978-1-4401-4960-3 (cloth)
ISBN: 978-0-595-61007-5 (ebk)

Printed in the United States of America.

DISCLAIMER

The purpose of this book is to educate. It is sold with the understanding that neither the publisher nor the author shall have neither liability nor responsibility for any injury caused or alleged to be caused by the information in this book. This book is not intended in any way to serve as a replacement for professional medical advice. Rather it is meant to encourage you, to use my experiences as an example of how to take responsibility for your own health with the aid of trained, certified healing professionals. I am telling my story, not rendering medical advice in any way. Throughout this book I encourage the reader to seek out the council of medical and nutritional professionals or "healing coaches". I am not a medical doctor and do not offer any medical advice. The US Federal Drug Administration has not reviewed or endorsed any of the content in this book. Please seek the advice of qualified healing professionals as part of any healing program.

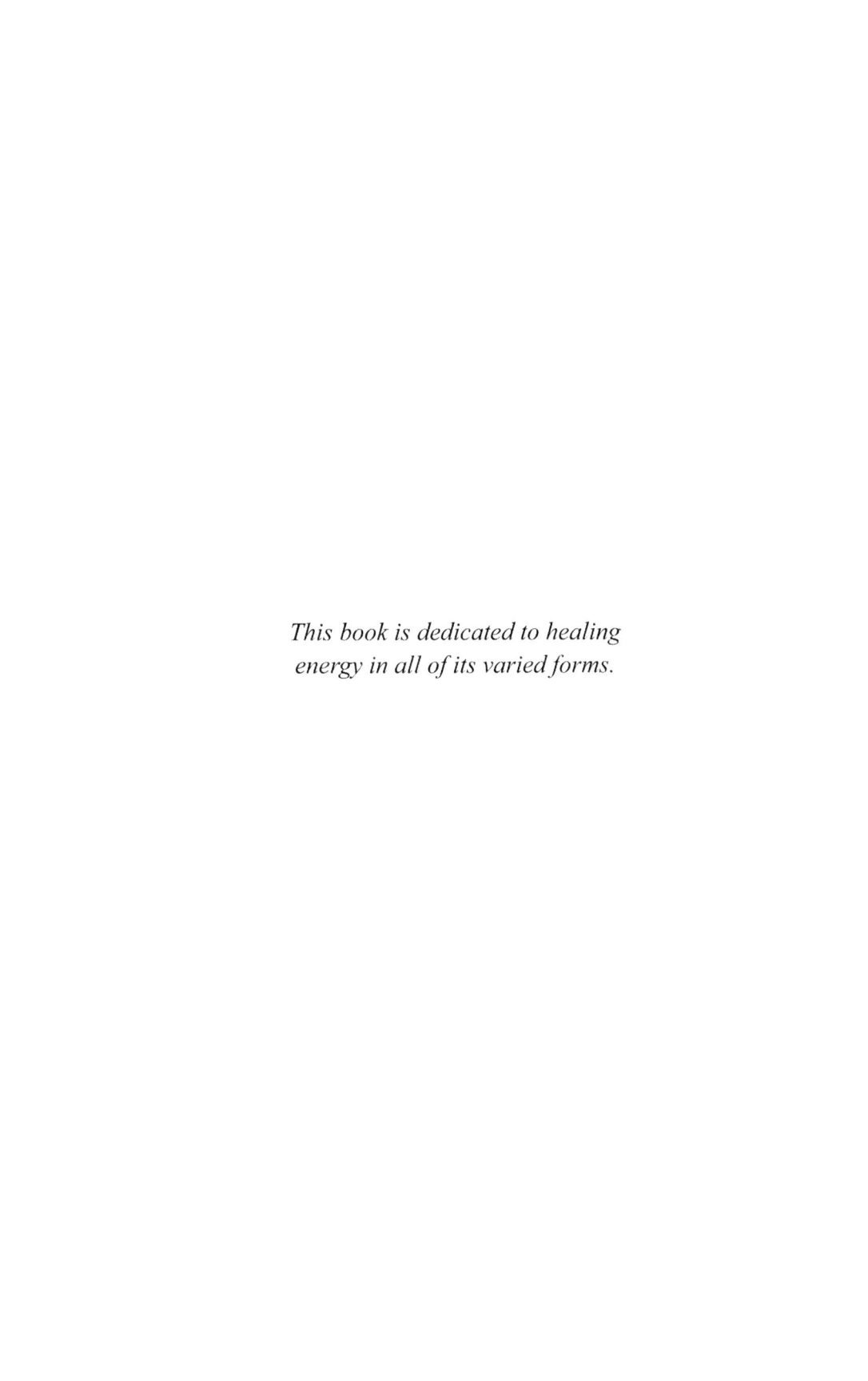

This book is dedicated to healing energy in all of its varied forms.

Contents

Acknowledgements xi

Foreword xiiii

Chapter 1 Introduction 1

Chapter 2 The Short List of My Most Powerful Discoveries 6

Section 1 Nutrition and Energy Food

Chapter 3 Healing Diets 19

Chapter 4 Vitamins & Supplements 47

Chapter 5 Herbs 64

Chapter 6 Internal Cleansing 71

Section 2 Energy Medicine—Moving Energy

Chapter 7 Acupuncture 91

Chapter 8 Acupuncture on Steroids 95

Chapter 9 Bio-Energetic Screening (Bio-Resonance Therapy) 104

Chapter 10 Emotional Freedom Technique Self-Administered
    Acupressure 110

Chapter 11 Massage Therapies 113

Chapter 12 Light and Color Therapy 116

Chapter 13 Crystals and Gems 128

Chapter 14 Radionics – Sending a Remedy through the Ether 137

Chapter 15 Effective Microorganisms™ – The Power of Magnetic Wave Resonance 151

Section 3 Two Healing Legends – Hazel Parcells & Edgar Cayce

Chapter 16 Dr. Hazel Parcells, PhD 159

Chapter 17 Edgar Cayce: The Sleeping Prophet 170

Section 4 Two Things of Immense Importance: Water and Your Mind

Chapter 18 Water as Healing Medicine 179

Chapter 19 The Mind/Body Connection 189

Section 5 Background Information

Chapter 20 My Story 205

Chapter 21 Your Present Medical Beliefs and How They Got There – The Flexner Report 224

Wrap Up *239*

Bibliography *242*

Website and Resources: www.richremedies.com *246*

About the Author *247*

Acknowledgements

This book has been a long time coming. There are many people who helped make this book a reality.

    Staring at a blank sheet of paper, searching for the words that create your story and writing a book can be a solitary, lonely effort. During this, my first writing journey, I free-associated with alot of people. Some I know and some are complete strangers who assisted me in countless ways. Thanks to everyone I met during this trip.

To the people I know:

First I would like to thank my lovely wife Linda who has endured several years of my self-discovery in the natural healing arena. The payoff was not obvious during the research/writing process for Rich Remedies Volume 1, but it will be some day. I am sure of this. Thanks for giving me the rope necessary to complete this important first step in my creative process and at times accepting what some might consider my "odd behavior" at times. It comes with the territory when you dare to think outside the box and challenge conventional wisdom.

    To my children: Emily, Christian, and Scott. If nothing else, I kept you laughing. This book was originally written for you as a short summary of my healing diaries, which spanned many years, and which I wanted to preserve for your benefit.... You got a whole book out of the deal. Please make use of this information.

    I love all of you.

Major contributors, guides, and supporters: Meridian Grace, ND, Colleen Reilly, Mikhail Teppone, M.D., and Terry Kast.

Many thanks to Joseph Dispenza, Dawson Church, Dr. Teruo Higa, William Two Feather and other authors/publishers who allowed me to reference their material on natural healing for this book.

Howard Tyson, my brother, proofread the manuscript and blazed the family book writing trail. Thanks for breaking the ice.

Janice Terra, who re-edited this book after reading the first issue because she believes in it.

Work mates who listened to my meandering, natural healing rants during the formulation of this book for a few years were: Jill Ford, Tom Brand, and Greg Stock. Appreciate you guys listening … whether you were interested or not … you politely listened. You kept me company during my solitary creative project. It helped immensely.…

Support Our Children – 10% of all author royalties are donated to The Austin Children's Shelter and the Make-A-Wish Foundation.

Writing a book is one of my life goals. Thanks. One down.… many books to go!

Foreword

The natural Healing adventures and discoveries of "Joe Six Pack"

"I am going to be and live healthy…just in time…Just before the chocolate pudding hits the fan, but not a day before."

"I'm going to lower my cholesterol…just in time…just before I hit the wall"

"I'm going to…just in time…"

This has been my internal thought process about health since I was a teenager and started having slight notions of my mortality. Have fun, run your body into the ground and quit just before your body starts to deteriorate. I am convinced by the way most people live that this thought process is quite common. It's been my way. This is the way of the character "Joe Six pack".

To me "Joe Sixpack" is the stereotypical American male who has a pretty basic, simple attitude about life and health. Give him a bag of chips, a hamburger, a few beers, a couch to lie on, and a sports event on television and he's set. Health and healing are the last thing on his mind. I haven't ever been this simple, naïve and lazy, but at times close. As long as something wasn't broken or painful, I typically ignored my health. When something did hurt, I very reactively went to the doctor and got my pills to fix the problem. Does this sound familiar?

After a few minor, but painful and inconvenient "warning" sicknesses, I adjusted my lifestyle slightly and changed my attitude concerning taking care of my health.

I made discoveries along the way that I thought would be useful to my children and maybe a few others. This book is not the same old wine in a new bottle; it is the best of the old wine mixed with the very best new wine, based on my experiences…a fine vintage for all time.

Here's how you will gain immediate value from what I have to say:

I have personally cured myself, naturally, of numerous sicknesses such as stomach ulcer, asthma, allergies, high cholesterol, food poisoning, and minor everyday health annoyances. After many trial and error attempts to get well, I have found some miraculous healing methods not in open view of the public because most people do not spend the time actively seeking, studying, and trying natural cures like I do. It's my "enlightened hobby" I guess, and a very useful one it is.

I stumbled and tripped over a few of them, completely by accident. More likely it is Divine Providence that I discovered them and am able to bring them to your attention in this book. Naturopaths may tell you that my information is "common" knowledge, in their circles, although I doubt it. Most of what you will find in the following pages is "uncommon knowledge" otherwise, we'd all be doing it. Wouldn't we?

You will get the benefit of my years of experience, avoiding a few mistakes which I have made, save lots of time/money and receive information on professional sources for healing.

My credentials

I am a seeker of truth and an advocate for my own personal health. As such, I have taken matters into my own hands on multiple occasions when conventional healthcare was not getting the job done.

Having an unconventional thirst for self-healing knowledge, I read a lot of stuff. Medical practitioners of many persuasions will skim through this book, writing me off as an uneducated, unqualified and uncertified amateur. I agree that I have very limited knowledge of anatomy, physiology, biology, and chemistry nor any clinical experience other than the healing work I have done on myself.

Academically I do not have the science background of some of the brilliant people in the practice of medicine. Yet, these same really "smart" people had no clue how to heal me without pumping me full of toxic chemicals. I got sicker and felt more pain using their "smart medicine."

In my circle of associates is a brilliant, accomplished neurosurgeon. He has produced many life saving medical innovations and saved many lives with his surgical techniques. He suffers from chronic asthma and allergies that have him on three separate inhalers and steroids which, in combination, are slowly killing him. I offered to lend him *Eat Right for Your Type* by Dr Peter D' Adamo, the blood type diet that contributed to healing my asthma and allergies. My friend politely declined my offer. His brilliant mind cannot accept a mental model that suggests that your blood type and diet can be a source of your cure. Coming from me, a pedestrian novice, was another problem I suspect. I also told him about cleansing and suggested that, over the years, all the medicine he has been taking had created a toxic state in his colon which was directly affecting the health of his lungs. He could not and would not accept my council because I am not a doctor. Who am I to give him advice? They were just suggestions. I don't give advice and I am not rendering any in this book.

One thing I have learned on this journey is that sage health advice and counsel comes from some of the most unlikely places. I have a natural knack for discovering healing things and an equally strong intuition for detecting frauds. Believe me, there are plenty of frauds in the "healthy living" arena.

I grew up thinking alternative healing and its practitioners were all nuts. Further, being a very skeptical person to begin with, selling me on this was not easy. I'm a tough sell when it comes to fads, new religions, off-center politics or other pre-fabricated cultural ideas presented by our mass media culture on a daily basis. My "BS meter" is very well calibrated. This new age stuff was hard for me to swallow for years. Some of it still is and I continue to find myself laughing out loud at some of the metaphysical stories I hear from the foo-foo crowd. Eventually, over time through experiencing dramatic healing results, I became a convert in some areas where I witnessed firsthand healing benefits.

I am probably just like many of you; born and raised on the sugar, refined food, meat and potatoes diet. I really had very little time for the "healthy" diet thing growing up and even into early adulthood.

I am not rendering advice in this book. I am not a licensed healthcare professional. I am just sharing my story and offering a few sign posts enabling you to find the path yourself. You can use what is in this book or reject it as you see fit. You will find what you need in your own time. But I guarantee that there are things in this book that can help you, a friend or a loved one, now or in the future. I have healed myself from multiple ailments over twenty years. I offer my experiences as an example of what is possible, but request that you find a competent healing coach or physician to direct your informed healing.

The patient who acts as her own doctor has a fool for a customer. Find a good healing coach. Trust me, I tried to treat myself for years and it's better to seek professional assistance when dealing with your health. It speeds things up and helps you avoid blind alleys and dead ends. I have run into my share.

I have a few secrets here and I am not just re-gifting health tips from all the usual, well-known sources. This is my story as an average person who went for medical treatment, but found out the hard way that the medicine I was getting, in certain cases, was making me worse. Instead of behaving like a helpless puppet, I took matters into my own hands, and cured myself. I won.

I advocate integrative medicine, i.e. combining allopathic and naturopathic medicine practices. You should be the master of your own destiny. Anyone who condemns any branch of healing is full of it. There is a place for all modes of healing, as long as they are used responsibly.

All schools of medicine work at some level, including the "placebo effect" where a patient is given a sugar pill, instead of real medicine, then gets better just because she believes she is better, even though the pill she is taking is a blank. This is the power of "Intention" which is: If you believe in the cure, you increase your chances of getting better tenfold. The placebo effect, although scorned by many in the medical establishment, is actually the most powerful natural remedy there is. There is nothing more powerful than your mind when it comes to healing yourself.

I now try to follow Benjamin Franklin's motto when it comes to my health:

> *"An Ounce of Prevention is Worth a Pound of Cure"*
> — Poor Richard's Almanac

- The best way to remain healthy is to stay out of the operating room.

- Being aware of what you are putting into your body at all times also contributes to this goal.

- Preventative health is more convenient, less time consuming and less painful than reactionary healthcare where you freak out because something has knocked you off your stride.

Some of Benefits of My Health Discoveries

Some of the powerful health discoveries in this book are not readily available to the general public or are obscured from public view because they are "unconventional".

What follows is a list of some of the things that I have learned throughout my journey. Naturally, your results will depend on the action you take.

- Slow and potentially reverse the aging process-naturally.

- You can heal yourself with the coaching of a natural physician.

- Learn about how I relieved an ulcer, allergies, lowered cholesterol, and chronic asthma after years of searching for natural remedies.

- There is hope for your recovery from illness…think out-of-the box with something new.

- Unconventional sources of information and treatments from experts in natural healing.

- Discover the secrets and techniques used by Soviet Sports Olympic medicine trainers in the 1970s to rapidly heal injuries incurred by their athletes, giving them a competitive edge. This same technique is healing a variety of ailments in people all over the world and you probably never heard of it. Well, now you will.

- A long distance healing technique that is unbelievable and miraculous. You have to read it to believe it!

- A plant-based nutriceutical I discovered that may fight some viruses, naturally, for a fraction of the cost of its synthetic cousin.

- Discover the magic of light and color.
- Effective Microorganisms EM™ – an incredible healing technology with multiple applications for healthy living.

Who should read this book?

- People who have tried the conventional medical treatments and want to learn more about alternative ways of healing. (I'm not advocating leaving your doctor, just get familiar with natural healing.)
- Anyone who is willing to take charge and responsibility for their own health.
- Athletes looking for a competitive edge.
- People who are just feeling tired and lousy and do not want to live this way.
- Those who want to lose weight in a sensible way anymore.

Life is about happiness and enjoyment. Get more of everything as you improve your health.

Let's face it; we're all going to pass from this physical plane of existence sometime. This is a given no matter how much we want to deny it, it's going to happen. What is important is the quality of your existence while you are here in this physi¬cal realm, which is directly proportionate to the quality of your health. It is harder to achieve this from a hospital bed or with an inhaler stuck in your mouth or a pocketful of pharmaceuticals, draining your wallet and your health.

Natural healing is here. It needs to be accessible and believable to mainstream people from someone who has tested many things and is a skeptic. I do not embrace most fads and I have an incredible BS meter built into my brain. This book is no BS.

I am a normal, fun loving person, not a monk. Like many of you,

I sometimes find the subject of holistic health and natural healing somewhat restrictive and stifling. There are so many "can't haves" in the clean, healthy living category that it becomes inconvenient and difficult to implement them in today's world. What I have found is life is full of compromises and contradictions, as are diets and wellness programs. I have discovered a variety of natural healing modalities that have worked for me in my own conflicted state. Some are mainstream and some are really far out. You pick and choose what works for you.

The key to being and staying healthy is listening to what your body is telling you and taking preventive measures before something becomes a full-blown disease. Most diseases take several years to develop so cutting them off at the pass before they gather strength is your best defense against them. The body replaces itself completely approximately every seven years. You can start today building a new body that will be completely different, and better seven years from now if you adopt healthy living habits.

May something here **resonate** with you and for you. It's all about **energy flow and the energetic frequencies** *that you encounter in your life at all levels. Once you understand this and manage them, you'll live a happier, healthier life.*

Check out this book, I think that you'll benefit from my healing journey.

— Richard

Chapter 1
Introduction

"Health" is energy flow. The free flow of energy through your physical, emotional and astral bodies determines your level of health. This was discovered by man thousands of years ago and is an irrefutable fact. This book, in its most basic premise, is to help you get your energy flowing through a variety of means.

"Disease" is the blockage of energy flow through your physical, emotional, and astral body. When a blockages occurs, bacteria, viruses, parasites, toxins and other invaders attack your body's weakened defenses resulting in illness.

Stick with me here. There is scientific proof of what I am saying.

These basic concepts have been applied in Traditional Oriental Medicine, by the ancient Egyptians and many indigenous populations worldwide. Man would never have evolved over 10,000 years had he not learned how to heal himself naturally. We'd all be gone had natural healing not been in existence since the beginning of time.

Again:

The fundamental cause of disease and all illnesses of a physical, mental and spiritual nature is **energy blockage**.

If you continue further, you will be shown ways to unblock your energy and heal yourself. This unblocking process takes many forms and techniques.

Understanding life energy (Ki) and putting it to proper use took me twenty years. (I'm kind of slow. I'm sure it won't take you as long to get and use energy.)

Everything in the Universe has a natural **resonance** and energy. Food, light, water, thoughts, feelings and emotions are all forms of energy. Humans and all matter are a vibrating, resonating mass of energy, simply vibrating at different rates.

This isn't my opinion, but scientific fact. We can see this phenomenon and measure it under high-powered microscopes. It is used in x-rays, CAT scans, biofeedback and Kirlian photography to detect and analyze the energy within the physical being.

All the concepts that are discussed in this book have an energetic effect in some way, shape, or form. So health and wellness comes down to Energy Management at its most basic form. In our human frame of reference and the way we have been conditioned to look at the world, the concept of energy management is foreign to most of us.

Meet Energy. It is Your Friend.

We are sources of light. Every cell, tissue and organ has its own specific radiation and produces its own specific magnetic field. These are now made use of in medicine for the diagnosis of illnesses. An example of this is Magnetic Resonance Imaging (MRI).

This conventional medicine technique is designed to measure the magnetic fields within our bodies. From this, three-dimensional images can be produced of all our inner organs which are considerably more accurate and precise than x-ray images. This is just one proof point that we really are all about energy.

Resonance is a concept that relates to everything in this book and explains how healing works. Each of us is a buzzing, swirling mass of atoms. We all have our own genetic makeup and DNA. Because of our unique, individual footprint, different things work to nourish and heal us at different times. Everyone is different. There is also a genetic individual predisposition towards diseases. So, to heal, you need to find energy sources that resonate with your individual physical, spiritual, mental, and emotional make up. This energy resonance streams from the universe through your subtle body, your physical body, into your organs, spine, blood, cells, and down into the molecules that make up your body.

We are holographic beings. This is a fancy term for saying "all for one and one for all". All parts of our physical being have intelligence and knowledge of all of the other parts. From your brain down to individual cells. One part relates and exchanges information with all the others. We are resonating, unified, whole beings. We are spiritual beings having a human experience.

Based on this concept, you should treat your mind, body and soul based on what is needed to make them whole and permit the smooth flow of energy. So when you look for the cure, whether it is vitamins, minerals, light, color, homeopathics, antibiotics or any other remedy, the right one is the one that resonates with your unique circumstances during a particular moment in your life.

I discovered and experienced this first hand through Radionics and with Biofeedback which are discussed later in this book.

Introduction 4

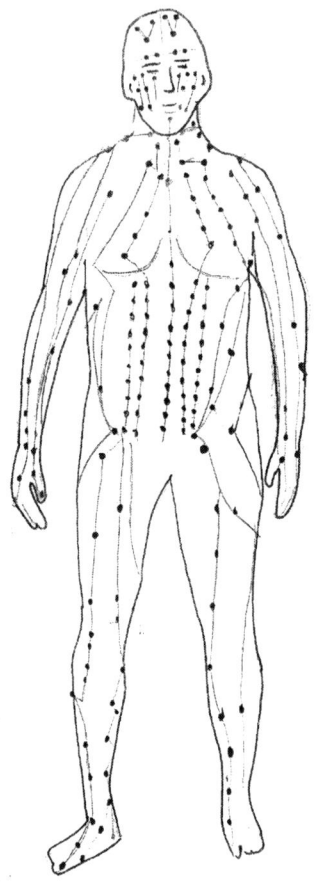

This is my illustration of the meridian system in the human body and the associated potent points. The meridians are the energy (Ki) highway that connects the skin, organs, and all body systems. By stimulating the potent points, it is said that a healer can stimulate the clearing of Ki or life energy in the body. This clearing of Ki opens the free flow of energy throughout the body according to Traditional Oriental Medicine. When Ki flows freely, we are healthy. Blocks of Ki are caused by emotional trauma, daily stress, spiritual crisis, chemical pollution, acidosis, heavy metal contamination, and other energy drains/blockages.

5   Rich Remedies

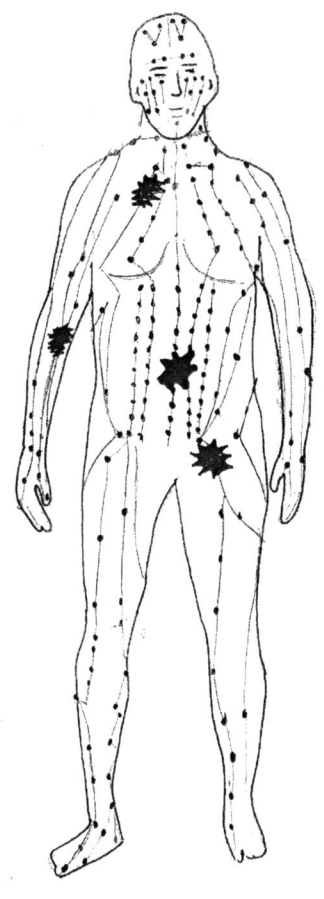

When life energy (Ki) blockages occur in the meridian system, disease often results. The blockage can be relieved in some cases by Acupressure, Acupuncture, Light Puncture, Emotional Freedom Technique, AcuScen, Radionics, and other energy moving solutions. Illnesses and blockages can sometimes be detected by Bio-Energetic Screening, Radethesia, and Bio-feedback technologies that measure the flow through the body's energetic system.

Chapter 2
The Short List of My Most Powerful Discoveries

I look at healing minor and major health issues like a good mechanic looks at repairing a car: start with the cheapest, smallest, easiest components (repairs) and work your way up the chain to the more expensive, intrusive procedures.

For example, if the electric window in my car won't open, the mechanic first replaces the fuse, and then he looks at the electrical connections and relays, checks the window switch, and, as a last resort, starts cutting cable and replaces the window motor. The irresponsible, rip-off mechanic goes to the shelf and replaces the window motor straight away for $550, when the fix could have been a simple five dollar switch or one dollar fuse. This has actually happened to me with an Audi that I once owned. Ouch! That was expensive! And painful! The same goes for your health. I start with a natural, cheap, nonintrusive remedy based upon the advice of my doctor and nutritionist.

Some medical doctors act like the bad mechanic. They will look at a person as a "sick organ" and remove that organ or prescribe massive amounts of toxic pharmaceuticals to "fix" the problem, when maybe all the patient needed was some internal cleansing, minerals and energy therapy; all inexpensive, benign, and non-intrusive treatments.

With physicians, I look for a doctor who listens to me and makes me part of the healing process; a facilitator, not a dictator. One who understands everything that is going on in my life, including my diet, occupation, stress-creating situations, living environment, family history, physical appearance, symptoms, and vital signs.

The best doctors then seek minimally intrusive, natural cures, such as medicinal herbs, vitamin or mineral supplementation, therapeutic massage, cleansing diets, detoxification, exercise and any other cost-effective, non-intrusive, non-toxic healing approaches. Then they counsel on the emotional or spiritual aspects of the person to flush out any other possible root causes of the illness, which in many cases are psychological in nature.

How many times has your doctor prescribed colloidal minerals, herbs, or an organic vegetable diet? This is rare. In my early years, I'd usually leave the Doc's office with a prescription for pills, whether I needed them or not.

This is not necessarily the doctor's fault. Some people actually feel cheated if they do not receive a prescription for drugs, as many of us have been conditioned to believe that our "fix" is in the pill.

Sometimes it is and many times it isn't, in my opinion.

Sickness can be rooted in life factors like an overbearing boss at work, an abusive relationship, a phobia such as fear of flying, a lack of self esteem, or any number of non-physical issues that manifest themselves as physical ailments. The goal in medicine should be to look at the whole person, not just the physical symptoms.

In my opinion, the last resort should be prescription of drugs or surgery, unless it is an emergency situation or readily apparent that a drug will expedite healing. Drugs are good if used appropriately. Today, they are way over-prescribed.

Like a good mechanic, the effective healer looks for the root cause of the illness, then finds the least expensive and intrusive method to address the problem, while allowing the body to heal itself.

> ### *My Mechanic's Checklist*
>
> √ Stress-related factors: Deal with the root cause
>
> √ Check for Vitamin and/or mineral deficiency
>
> √ Internal system condition: Check for presence of heavy metals, parasites, yeast, or accumulated toxins

Here is a summary of the wonderful things that I've learned that may be of help after you have consulted your naturopathic doctor or nutritionist:

Emotions are the root cause of 85% of diseases

Based on observation, stress produced by early childhood traumas, business pressure, pressure to succeed, poverty, tribal beliefs, and mental depression, are the major causes of disease. If you believe in reincarnation, then past life stress and karmic lessons play into this as well. Many people do not believe in reincarnation so if you don't, scratch this one. Stress weakens the body enabling disease to take root. Stress, at its most basic level, is the fight or flight syndrome that is continually at work between your brain, adrenal glands, heart, and every cell in your body. It's your mind and/or body's basic survival mechanism. It is continually processing information and reacting to it through thought and chemical responses. If these responses are negative, the result is toxic to your body.

Emotions are seemingly difficult and evasive things to deal with because they are so deeply ingrained in us and the solution really needs to come from within. Our tendency is to look outside ourselves for the answer. There are tools, such as meditation, light therapy, EFT, radionics, as well as a number of other natural remedies that may provide relief. The power of your own Intentions is probably the best tool. It all comes down to moving energy in its many forms which is really the underlying message of this entire book. Often times: "It's not what you eat. It's what is eating you."

Lipid Exchange Therapy

This has amazing, miraculous potential. I recently started incorporating Lipid Exchange Therapy into my dietary regiment with the use Phosphatidylcholine (PC), a 4:1 ratio of Omega 6 and Omega 3 fatty acids. PC has been found to improve the conditions of patients with **Alzheimer's, Bipolar Disorder, Amyotrophic Lateral Sclerosis (ALS or Lou Gehrig's Disease)), Multiple Schlerosis (MS), Lyme Disease, Chronic Fatigue Syndrome, Fibromyalgia, Autism, MS, Hepatitis C, cardiovascular disease, Parkinson's** and many more.1 I use it as a preventative measure to aid me in heading off the onset of some of the diseases I have listed here. Will it work? I have no clue, but doing nothing is not an option. Stay tuned. An ounce of prevention is worth years in assisted living for me. (See Chapter 4)

Get Alkaline

Acidosis plays a central role in disease and aging. Highly acidic body fluids are breeding grounds for all illnesses. A simple way to counteract these effects is to get your fluids more base (pH 7.0 or higher). There is way too much acid in the Western diet. Animal protein and fast foods are the biggest culprits. I have seen astonishing healing results in people who get their pH to 7.0 or above. I have been using a sink-top water ionizer and have seen improvements in my alkaline level as measured by the litmus paper test. Ionized water detoxifies the body and has contributes to improving health over all.(See Chapter 19.)

Effective Microorganisms EM™

Effective Microorganisms EM™ were discovered in 1982 in Japan by Dr. Teruo Higa, a horticulturalist, during his research into finding natural alternatives to chemical fertilizers. They are amazing beneficial bacteria with applications in human health, agriculture, waste management, water purification, construction, and many other uses. I have used the health/nutrition products, garden products, and ceramics. These are truly amazing products that exhibit an energetic frequency known as magnetic wave resonance, which have been found to enhance beneficial life forms wherever they are introduced. (See Chapter 15)

The Neural-arc Reflex

This is the discovery made by Dr. Bernard Jensen that the bowel is connected to nerves and organs in every part of your body. If your bowel is upset, infected and/ or clogged, the neurologically connected part of your body will be affected.2 This phenomenon is known as "referred pain."

Over 70% of disease originates in the gut. Clean it up and you will realize incredible health and vitality. The colon is the starting point of most disease. If you care for your colon, with proper nutrition, cleansing, and a calm emotional state, you have a high probability of avoiding most diseases. There seems to be an epidemic of colitis, irritable bowel syndrome, spastic colon, and colon cancer in this country. Name just about any other disease and it has some connection to the health of your colon ... (See Chapter 9.)

Detoxification

In our society, detoxification is associated with treating drug addicts and alcoholics, which it often is. But, the major beneficial application is really to help make healthy people healthier. The human body has a tremendous ability to fight any discase or allergy, if it is free of large quantities of toxins. A cell can live almost indefinitely, if the

---

1   Haverford Wellness Center Website, www.haverfordwellnesscenter.com/about

fluids surrounding it are clean and nourishing. If you live in a major industrial city and eat the standard American diet, you are most likely toxic and in need of cleansing. Many of our bodies are so polluted with chemicals and waste products that our immune systems are no longer capable of fighting disease. One of the basic, funda¬mental causes of illnesses is auto-intoxication (self pollution). Purging your body of toxic chemicals and heavy metals, which are everywhere in industrial societies, will help cure many allergies and diseases by restoring health to the blood and organs.

Fasting is a form of detoxification that is practiced by all of the major religions of the world on holy days. I fast on a liquid food diet and vitamin supplements three to four times a year, four to five days each time, to give my body a rest from solid food. This is a great way to detoxify the body. Digesting food consumes a tremendous amount of your life energy. By fasting, you enable the body to focus on repairing and restoring its health, naturally.

There is a school of thought that says we could all live to over one hundred years of age if we ate just one (1) nutritious meal per day, instead of the typical three.

Glycemic Index

Consciously monitoring your Insulin Response by eating low carbohydrate foods is perhaps the most effective way to lose weight, reduce your chances of diabetes, cancer, and just about every disease. All diseases and parasites use sugar as fuel. It's all about managing glucose (sugar) in your diet and body. Many good things spring from getting sugar, in its many forms, out of your diet.3 (See Chapter 3 Healing Diets.)

Light Therapy

Phototherapy has been used for patients with chronic fatigue syndrome, irregular menstrual problems, thyroid difficulties, insomnia, and depression. Light therapy affects the human energetic system the same way as acupuncture and chiropractic treatments do. I have used light therapy in rudimentary ways for a number of things. Because that we are "light beings" I believe it has had a beneficial effect. (See Chapter 12. Light and Color Therapy)

The Miracle Mineral

According to Dr Norman Shealy, MD, PhD, and other natural healing experts, many illnesses are related in some way to a magnesium deficiency in the body. This common "dirt mineral" governs a lot of bodily processes including metabolism, calcium absorption, mood, sleep, and muscular function. According to Dr. Shealy, a vast majority of the population of the United States has a deficiency in magnesium and would benefit from supplementation. I get most of my magnesium from the vegetables grown in my garden. My garden soil is liberally fertilized with magnesium sulfide aka Epsom salts. I eat alot of leafy green veggies and, when traveling, I take magnesium supplements to insure that I get enough of this important, life-sustaining mineral.

The Blockbuster Anti-Aging Tonic- Vivix™

This is a discovery of mine that was added to this book at the last minute due to its awesome healing potential. Vivix™ is a patented cellular anti-aging tonic made from grape extracts that are known to naturally contain massive amounts of the ant-aging compound resveratrol and polyphenols that were developed over years of development by Shaklee Corporation. (See Chapter 3. Vitamins and Supplements)

Sleep

The amount of sleep your body needs varies from person to person. Eight hours of sleep is the standard, but there are people who can

---

2   Jensen, Dr. Bernard. *Dr. Jensen's Guide to Better Bowel Care.* New York: Avery, Penguin Putman, 1999, p86

get by perfectly on less than five. Sleep deprivation impacts mental clarity, alertness, reaction time, immune system function, heart function and a host of other bodily functions. (I personally need at least six hours to function effectively.) Sleep disorders have a huge negative impact on all facets of your health. Your body repairs itself while you sleep.

Light therapy and magnesium supplementation are two things that can help you get back your ZZZs if you suffer from insomnia.

Color

It took me 49 years to find this one. Color? Yes, it's a fundamental part of life. Get it through fresh vegetables or in a rainbow-colored salad. Red, yellow orange, green blue, purple, and white vegetables mixed, will provide your body with the full spectrum of colors it needs. Get sunlight. You can also get color through "rainbow water" which is discussed in Chapter 14.

Find Yourself a Healing Coach

I have worked with a number of great allopathic and naturopathic healers. Before you do anything to treat a disease, find a physician or healer who embraces all modalities of healing. This can be an enlightened MD, a holistic doctor, or naturopathic physician. When you find a good physician, be a co-pilot in your diagnosis and treatment. They are only your coach. You are responsible for the cure. For a directory of physicians in your area contact the **American Holistic Medical Association** (PO Box 2016, Edmonds, WA 98020; Phone: 425-967-0737; Fax: 425-771-9588; e-mail: INFO@holisticmedicine.org).

Nutritionists

Find a clinically trained, degreed nutritionist to aid you in your

---

3   *Canadian Diabetes Association. http://www.diabetes.ca/*

health plan. This is tricky because there are a lot of people who have a nutritionist degree, but don't really know what they are talking about. You can get a correspondence course degree off of the back of a bubble gum wrapper and claim to be a nutritionist. A starting place for names is your local health food store or contact the **American Dietetic Association** (120 S. Riverside Plaza, Suite 2000, Chicago, Ill. 60606; Member Services Phone: (312)-877-1600 ext4864; website: www.eatright.org). I tried to do all of this healing stuff on my own, and have confirmed that the least successful patient acts as his own doctor. Get a trained, qualified healing coach.

Your cure: Nothing works the same way for everyone. Every body, mind, and soul has a unique blueprint that has to be matched with the correct cure. We have different genes, ancestors, tribal beliefs, environments, climates, magnetic earth fields, life experiences, blood types, and other unique characteristics that make global recommendations for cures impossible. There are general rules of thumb that can be applied to everyone. Find the ones that work (resonate) for you.

Meditation: Like fasting, all of the great prophets practiced meditation in order to get in touch with their spirit and to heal their soul, as well as their body. Tap into the mind/body connection. I do this for between 5 and 20 minutes daily. The benefits cross all categories of mind/body/spirit healing and are too numerous to list here. I am a novice in the scheme of things here, but the little meditation I do is a big help in all aspects of my life. Researchers at Harvard University have found that meditation can prolong life in the elderly. Doctors in England found that diet, exercise, and the practice of stress-reduction techniques, of which meditation is the most important, can actually reverse coronary disease.

Exercise: Excercise at least 20 minutes, five days per week. Get off your caboose and get moving. It does not matter what you do, just do it. Everyone has 20 minutes. Walk the extra five blocks to work, park at the furthest end of the Wal-Mart parking lot. Take the stairs instead of the elevator, walk to the corner store, and find opportunities in your daily schedule to elevate your heart beat. Exercise is right next to meditation on my list of high priority daily activities. It helps with circulation, metabolism, glucose processing, oxygen-intake- to name just a few benefits.

Give: Give your time to others. I participate in community service and volunteer work. It is actually more beneficial to me than to the people I am trying to help. Giving is the opposite, but complementary end of, receiving. I have gotten healthier since I started rendering service to those in need. It only requires a few hours per week. Like meditation and exercise, giving to others is an integral part of my personal wellness regimen on a weekly basis.

Try this for your own health and well being, it really works.

Energy Flow ("The flow of life"): Everything in life has its own frequency, flow and natural rhythm. In humans you are healthy when your thoughts, emotions, fluids, electricity, food, and energies are flowing freely. When there is a blockage of any kind, disease ensues. Energy flow (Ki) - energy in all of its forms, electricity, light, thoughts, nutrients, and other energies needs to be flowing. Dam this natural flow and you create disease. Everything in this book deals with energy in one way or another since we are energetic beings. There are a variety of terms this life energy: Ki, Qi, Chi, and Prana, all meaning life force.

Skim through this book right now and find one thing that you think you can easily do and do it. It can be as simple as fixing the water that you drink and installing a water filter in your house or understanding at a basic level the glycemic index and then reducing high glycemic foods in your diet, like refined sugar. Or, if you're really brave, cleanse yourself and see how much better you feel.

I do not live like a monk and do not expect anyone else to either. My intention is to provide insights into different levels of well-being and useful information that will enhance the quality of your life based on my experience. It took me years of trial and many errors. I am still not finished with my project.

Here's years of experience bottled into a couple hours of reading. You decide what works for you, what you will actually commit to, and what you can afford. Any improvement, however small, is a step in a positive direction. I am happy, healthy, and at peace with myself. It takes a little effort, but it is worth the price.

The journey of 1,000 miles starts with the first step. Take it!

SECTION 1
NUTRITION AND ENERGY FOOD

Chapter 3
Healing Diets

"Make food thy medicine and medicine thy food."
— Hippocrates

Sources of high energy food

The best source for energy food? Local, organic, and free range "slow food."

Before venturing into healing diets -I want to talk about food that heals. My experience is that if you consume locally grown (within 150 miles from where you live) natural, fresh, unprocessed foods and drink pure, clean water, you have locked in over half of the secrets to healthy living. Mass marketed supermarket foods (non-organic) often contain pesticides, chemical fertilizer residues, and bacteria such as salmonella.

Food that heals and vitamins

Fresh, local organic, minimally processed food is the best source of nutrition. I make an effort to buy organic, locally grown produce, when possible, at local farms, farmers' markets, and food co-ops. This is by far the best way to get nutrition. If you can do this, you need very little in the way of vitamin supplementation. The exceptions to additional supplementation are digestive enzymes and probiotics. These, in my opinion, are mandatory, no matter how well you eat, as they are not available from vegetables.

There is an argument that our modern farming practices have depleted the soil of minerals and, as a result, our food is deficient in nutritional value. To make up for this shortfall we must take vitamins and minerals. I subscribe to this theory, if you do not have access to fresh, organic produce. I also believe that you need vitamin supplementation when you have a deficiency that is causing health problems. This is where a nutritionist comes in. If you are in good health I think there is a case to be made for reducing your vitamin and/or mineral expenditures.

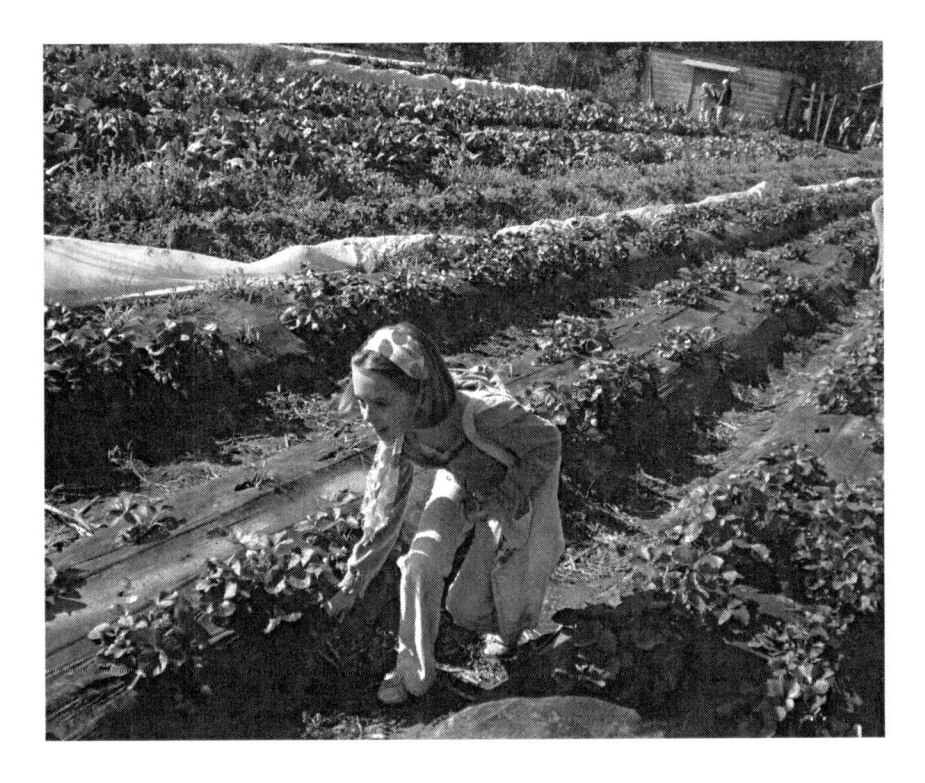

This is my daughter Emily picking fresh, organic strawberries at Boggy Creek Farm in Austin, Texas. We buy most of our produce from local area organic farms. This supports the family farm, provides us with nutritious, chemical free food, and is the best tasting food you will ever eat. If you have access to local, organic food, you need very little in the way of nutritional supplementation unless you have a diagnosed vitamin/mineral deficiency as this food

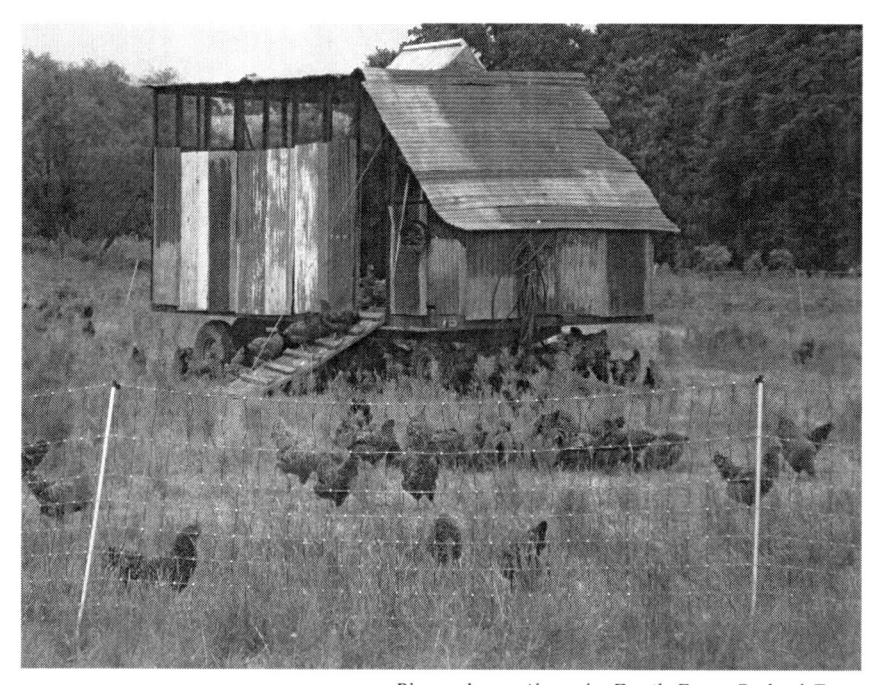

Photo taken at Alexander Family Farm, Garland, Texas

Grass fed, free range, organic chickens. This is "slow food". Poultry raised the old fashioned way before the advent of factory farms.

These chickens are moved weekly in their mobile chicken condominium to fresh pasture where they are free to peck away at grass, worms, insects, and anything else that nature provides. They are "happy and healthy chickens". The chickens and eggs taste great and are good for you. No growth hormones or anti-biotics are fed to these chickens.

Factory farm chickens are raised inside giant buildings with thousands of other chickens. They are fed antibiotics, growth hormones, sometimes arsenic, and are confined to tiny cages. They are "stressed out" chickens. You ingest all of these hormones, chemicals, and stress when you eat factory farm chickens. In most places, this is all that is available for purchase. Most of the chicken you get in markets and restaurants are raised in this unhealthy, inhumane way.

Go free range, organic if you can. We buy local, organic food every chance we get.

Macrobiotics

In my 20s I discovered macrobiotics and healed a very painful stomach ulcer. The term "Macrobiotics" has always been a turn-off for me because it sounds kind of weird and spacey, but in substance it is phenomenal. Why don't they just call it "the best healing diet in the world?" It is a very healthy way to live.

In Greek macro means "great" and bios means "life." It does produce a great life. The trick is not to get over-the-top weird like some macros I've met. Some are the most dull, anally retentive, and fearful people on the planet. Some won't eat food prepared in a pan previously used to cook meat. The way I look at it, if the pan has been washed thoroughly, it should be fine to use to cook vegetables. You can go off the deep end with this diet.

Back in my 20s, with an ulcer burning a hole through my stomach and my faith in conventional medicine waning, I decided that I needed to take responsibility for my own healing. I came across a book that caught my attention, changed the way I looked at health and healing and, in many ways, changed my perspective on life itself. The book was *Natural Healing Through Macrobiotics* by Michio Kushi.

Macrobiotics, the ancient art of health and longevity, has been hidden from most of the world's population for centuries. When I found this book I felt like the French soldiers who found the Rosetta stone in 1799. The book was inspiring! It opened my eyes to truths about health and healing that not only made sense, but were completely new to me. Additionally, it brought home the fact that nat¬ural healing has been obscured from view by ignorance, the medical commu¬nity, and commercial interests that make money off bad food and sometimes bad medicine.

The term "Macrobiotic" sounds odd and sterile, but it covers a way of looking at the whole cycle of life, as well as our relationship to the Universe. It is a holistic view of the world and our place in it, not just a diet that espouses getting into rhythm with nature in all aspects of our lives. Although a very difficult thing to accomplish in our busy industrial society, it is a worthy goal nonetheless.

Kushi's book links the Order of the Universe with the basic principles of diet, food, health, and life itself. At the core of the process is the harmony of opposites, keeping yin and yang properly balanced and removing energy blockages. The key concepts from this body of work that resonated most with me and led me to the ultimate kernel of truth about diet and health were the following:

- The quality of your blood determines the quality of your cells, immune system, thoughts, and the overall condition of your body and spirit. Like koi swimming in a pond, your surrounding water determines the quality of your health.

- Acid kills. Foods with an alkaline pH (between 7.0 and 10) should be consumed and foods with a pH of less than 5.0 should be reduced and/or avoided when possible.4 A diet of whole grains, beans, and vegetables should be consumed for maximum health. There are alkaline drinks and supplements that can help neutralize the unhealthy acidic things we consume. I will cover these later for those who cannot follow the restricted dietary regimen of the macrobiotic diet.

Macrobiotic Foods—High-Level Summary Guidelines[5]

Grains	40 to 60 percent daily*
Vegetables	25 to 30 percent daily
Beans	5 to 10 percent daily
Soups	5 to 10 percent daily
Sea vegetables	3 to 5 percent daily

Beverages	According to thirst
Condiments	Special vegetarian varieties
Pickles	Small amounts
Fish	0 to 3 times per week
Fruit	2 to 3 times per week
Desserts	Unbleached flour, no refined sugar. 2 times per week
Nuts, seeds	Daily
Sweeteners	0 to 3 times per week. Rice and barley syrup preferred.

*Note: This is the macrobiotic diet recommendation that I followed twenty years ago. I do not subscribe to this any longer and believe that much lower amounts of grains and all carbohydrates should be consumed. Your food should be fresh, minimally processed and, preferably, organic. It is also recommended that you eat locally grown produce that is in season.

Animal protein, a staple of many Western diets, is eliminated or substantially reduced in macrobiotics. Refined sugar, flour, factory processed foods, and artificial ingredients are avoided.

Nightshade plants, such as eggplant, tomatoes, and potatoes, are to be avoided or minimized if you are sick, as well as other "tropical foods."[1] These are said to cause arthritis and reduce the immune system's function in temperate climates making us more susceptible to colds and influenza. If you look, you will see no nightshades served in macrobiotic restaurants.

I recommend that you pick up a few of the books listed in the Bibliography and visit a macrobiotic restaurant when you have a chance. I admit that this is a pretty superficial attempt to cover a huge area, but I'm just here to point the way.

---

4 Kushi, Mishio, and Alex Jack. *The Book of Macro-Biotics*. New York & Tokyo: Japan Publications, 1986, pp122–125

My Experience

The reality is that this diet is very hard to follow, but in many of its tenets can easily be incorporated into your daily life.

In a perfect world I could eat a macrobiotic diet with a few minor modifications. I like meat and eat it 1 or 2 times per week. I tried macrobiotics for a few months, cured the stomach ulcer, and felt great. I did gain a few pounds because of all the brown rice I ate every day and I also felt like I had to eat twice the amount of food to feel satiated. The problem was that I travel on business and hang out with people who are carnivores. I also found that my diet was inconveniencing and alienating some people. They looked at me with suspicion, like I was some bohemian oddball who was practicing a "hippie diet". Not that I permit other people's opinions to rule my life, but food and meals can be great unifiers or separators of people. I don't like unnecessary separation. There were also aspects of life, like partying, that I wasn't willing to give up. When the thing that you are doing to make yourself better starts to cause stress and inconvenience, you shift gears, find a happy medium, and compromise.

The Macrobiotic Diet set the stage for an awareness of the healing potential of the body. It gave me the capacity to understand the consequences of consuming certain foods (cause and effect). I noticed a change in the way I felt, physically and mentally, after I ate certain foods and knew I had a safety net of the Macrobiotic Diet to fall back on should I get sick.

I highly recommend that people who are feeling bad or have an illness investigate this diet. Use macrobiotics in combination with the Blood Type Diet, discussed in the next section, for better results.

The dietary regimen I fell back into after macrobiotics was a 75% vegetarian to 25% meat diet, i.e., 75% of the food I consumed

---

5   Ferre, Carl. *Macrobiotics. Crossing Press, Berkely, Ca. 1997.pp15–16.*

was vegetable or grain-based and 25% contained animal fat (meat, dairy, fish, poultry, and eggs). My personal formula also incorporated rawer, uncooked food, such as salads, than the standard macrobiotic diet recommends. The 75% vegetarian to 25% omnivore ratio is my personal preference since it fits well with my travel, business, family, and other variables that limit one's capability to follow a strict dietary regimen, incorporation of some of the concepts from the Blood Type Diet (which follows).

Check out any book by Michio Kushi and George Osawa, the patron saints of macrobiotics. Also see the *The Okinawa Program*, a Harvard University study published in 2003 that discusses the longevity of the people who live on the island of Okinawa, Japan. There is a high concentration of 100+ year old people who eat a macrobiotic diet living there. Interestingly, cancer and heart disease, the two main killers in America, are virtually unknown amongst this population. Additional factors that play into this high centenarian population are reduced stress, strong family units, spirituality, and some genetics. However, there is definite irrefutable medical proof from Harvard University that the greatest contributor to their health and longevity is their macrobiotic diet.

Note: Through additional research and experimentation, I have concluded that the Macrobiotic Diet includes too many grains for my personal body and blood type; therefore, I have substantially reduced my consumption of grains and beans from what is recommended. My reason for doing this is to improve my insulin response and blood sugar levels, as I have a very slight diabetic tendency which I have chosen to reduce through my conscious reductions in carbohydrates. It's a personal choice made based on my own individual situation. Green leafy vegetables and high quality proteins are my dietary mainstays at this time.

---

1   Kushi, Mishio, and Alex Jack. *The Book of Macro-Biotics*. New York & Tokyo: Japan Publications, 1986, pp119–221

Blood Type Diet

I recommend that you visit your local public library and check out a copy of Dr. Peter J. D'Adamo MD, *Eat Right for Your Type* to get the details about this interesting diet.

Since I began this diet, I've spoken with a number of doctors and nutritionists who say that 90% of the benefits of this diet can be found in sound nutritional practices that are not necessarily tied to your blood type. By avoiding highly processed foods, sugars, hydrogenated oils, and most of the things that are passed off as "nutritional" by the fast food industry, you can improve your health dramatically. I will tell you about my experience with the Blood Type Diet at the end of this section. It provided me with the sound nutritional guidelines that I needed during a chronic illness and I think it is an interesting spin on food. Bottom line-cut down on animal fat, wheat, peanut products, hydrogenated oils, dairy, and grain-fed meats and you will improve your health.

Dr. D'Adamo is a naturopathic physician, researcher, and anthropologist all wrapped into one. He has studied the history of man, our evolution, tribal migrations, and the environments that mandated certain diets and, by extension, evolved our blood types over centuries. Basically he determined that we are what we have historically eaten over the centuries of evolution. It makes sense. Man's body, cells, and genes adapted over time to the foods that were readily available.

According to his research, how our digestive tracts, metabolisms, and immune systems developed over time is reflected in our blood types. Naturally, when you wander off of your historic diet, your body reacts. This is especially true when the foods that you consume are highly processed and vastly different from your historical roots. With a supply chain of foods from everywhere on the globe, plus hyper-processing, our bodies don't always recognize what we are eating as food.

As you probably know, there are four blood types. Each has its own unique characteristics that are explained in detail in *Eating Right for Your Type*. Here is a very simplistic summary of the characteristics[2]: Type O (my blood type) should eat a low carbohydrate diet and some meat. O Type blood is the universal donor for blood transfusions. Type A blood types are best suited to vegetarian diets and minimal animal fats. Type B's can eat a varied diet that includes meat and dairy. Type AB shares the characteristics of both A and B.

The key discovery for me, and the one that facilitated a miraculous healing event in my life, was the understanding of antigens and lectins. This was a critical missing piece in the puzzle to conquer my debilitating allergies. It is also an important piece for you to understand, so read this quickly.

"Antigens" are chemical markers found in the cells of our bodies that have the ability (intelligence) to detect the unique chemical "fingerprints" of everything into which they come into contact. They serve as cellular antibodies or gate guards against invading viruses and bacteria. Each blood type has its own unique antigens which is why we have four types and why you need to have blood types matched prior to a blood transfusion. If you mix incompatible blood types, you will have a battle of antigens and a major bad reaction (death). This same battle occurs with certain foods that you consume.

"Lectins" are proteins found in foods having properties that affect your blood and interact with your blood type antigens.[3]

Understanding the connection between blood type antigens and the reactions that they were having with the lectins in food created an "ah ha" moment for me. The antigens attack incompatible lectins like they attack invading bacteria and viruses! Viola! Allergies = the battle of Lectins vs. Antigens! Some foods resonate better with your antigens than others.

Since reading the book I have discussed this with a number of healing professionals who have all had differing opinions about this diet and how universally it can be applied to people.

One healing professional told me that natural foods, especially raw foods in combination with digestive enzymes, will provide relief to allergy suffers and improve health in general.

The body knows what to do. We just have to give it the tools (right foods) to get the job done. I have yet to find a supplement that actually out performs Mother Nature in the long haul. Diet and nutrition will always be the foundation that vibrant health is built on.

My Experience

For about ten years I was pretty faithful to the 75% vegetables and 25% protein diet I had created for myself based on some of the things learned in macrobiotics. There were occasional lapses but, in general, I was compliant. I noticed as I got into my 40s that my allergies were getting progressively worse. They must be cumulative, because every year of my life the discomfort associated with seasonal allergies increased.

Then, in 2000, I moved to Leesburg, Virginia from Pennsylvania. There was construction excavation in our neighborhood with dirt flying everywhere, plus a lot of cedar trees (actually juniper) in the area. Mold was also very bad in this area. My allergies flared up to the point where I contracted asthma. It was especially bad from November through February when the cedar trees pollinated. I went from running 5 miles per day to 2 miles then to riding my bicycle because my breathing became so constricted from allergies. I will add stress to this asthma equation because it was also a contributing factor.

I had acupuncture administered and took Chinese herbs which seemed to reduce the symptoms a little, but did not completely eliminate them.

During this time I decided that it was time for a change of scenery and moved to Austin, Texas, the allergy capital of the world.

---

2   D'Adamo, Dr. Peter J. and Catherine Whitney. *Eating Right 4 Your Type.* New York: G.P. Putnam's Sons, 1996. pp 5 to 28. Note: *I focused my attention on the basic blood*

On brief business trips prior to moving to Austin, I had experienced very mild allergies symptoms but did not factor it into my relocation considerations.

Within two months of moving to Austin I developed severe asthma due to high levels of mold and pollen in the air. The conditions had me short of breath, wheezing, coughing, and expelling the most awful looking glue-thick, green gunk from my lungs. Sleep was impossible for more than a few hours before I would wake up coughing and expelling that gunk from my lungs. It felt as if the sickness had a personality of its own. Ask any allergy sufferer from Austin and they will support this story.

The asthma required several treatments with antibiotics, an inhaler, and a prescription for steroids as an anti-inflammatory for my lungs. Several people told me that my allergic reaction to the air in Austin was very common and to "get used to it." The doctor who was treating me told me that my regimen of antibiotics, steroids, and inhaler was going to be with me for a long, long time. The alternative was to go to an allergist, get pinpricked with a sample of common allergens, and then have injections of a serum that would enable my immune system to better tolerate pollens and molds. A mold injection, a cedar injection, a live oak serum injection, and who knows what else on a weekly basis? I hate shots and needles, so this was never really an option. Further, there was no guarantee that these expensive, inconvenient, and painful injections would even work.

All my life I have been blessed with good health. Being sick is not my natural state or one for which I have patience. Prescription drugs and conventional medicine were never part of my regimen either. The side effects of the prescriptions I was taking for the allergies were almost as bad as the asthma. The antibiotics screwed up my digestive tract and gave me diarrhea. (They disrupt the good bacteria in your intestines while they fight the bad bacteria that

---

3   D'Adamo, Dr. Peter J. and Catherine Whitney. *Eating Right 4 Your Type*. New York: G.P. Putnam's Sons, 1996 pp 5 to 28.

settle in your lungs.) Steroids upset my stomach making it feel like I had an ulcer. The inhaler had some stimulating chemical, like an amphetamine, in it that made me jumpy, irritable, and tense.

The prospect of being wed to this discomfort, to make me "better," was unacceptable, so I decided to take my care and recovery into my own hands. I chose not to accept the advice of my doctor (to get married to this semi-annual torture for the rest of my life). I know people who are hooked on inhalers and drugs for allergies and asthma. This wasn't going to be me! I took action.

First, I considered moving away from Austin: not a viable option since my family was settled in and I had become attached to this great city.

The second consideration was to find a natural, sustainable, drug-free way to fight the allergies. I chose this route.

I got the name of a local acupuncturist from an acquaintance of ours whose allergies had been treated with miraculous results. She had grown up in Austin with no allergies. However, after the age of 35 she developed chronic allergies. Doctors had tried serum injections of common allergens and then, when these did not work, gave her increasingly larger doses of steroids that eventually gave her a severe toxic reaction. As a last resort my friend went to an acupuncturist who cleared up her allergies within months. She never took another steroid or other medication for allergies. Acupuncture works miraculously for some people.

I was treated with acupuncture ten times and prescribed Chinese herbs that are thought to have medicinal effects for treating allergies and asthma. The acupuncturist also recommended the book *Eating Right 4 Your Type*.

The acupuncture treatments were invigorating and gave me a sense of well being, but did not stem the effects of the allergies. After my second treatment I suffered a "healing crisis" whereby the body gets worse before it gets better. The symptoms of the healing crisis were severe sinus headache, mild nausea, cramps, and sweating. It felt like the flu. The acupuncturist informed me that based on the healing crisis, my body was turning the corner on the allergies and that the treatments were working. I was told to be grateful for this agony. It was horrible!

Weeks went by with only a slight improvement in my condition. Unfortunately, in the ninth and second to last week of my acupuncture, I had a significant relapse and found myself back on antibiotics, the inhaler, and steroids. Very, very disheartening. Thoughts of moving from Austin came back to me as I could not deal with the thought of bi-annual suffering and pharmaceutical treatments that were as bad as the ailment itself. I felt like I was suffering from the flu all the time. It was awful!

The final straw occurred while on a trip to Manhattan in early January. I woke up coughing at 2:00 am on successive mornings, unable to sleep without the assistance of my inhaler. My body was weak, my head ached from the constant coughing, I was tired, and my asthma was getting worse.

Upon my return to Austin I scanned the yellow pages for naturopathic doctors. I was able to secure the last appointment, at 6:00 pm, with a local naturopath I was their last patient of that day. After a brief examination by the doctor, I had a consultation with a nutritionist who prescribed, in addition to Chinese herbs, magnesium, omega-3 fatty acids, and vitamin C, natural anti-inflammatories, as well as the book *Eating Right 4 Your Type*. This was the same book that the acupuncturist had recommended six months prior and was still collecting dust on my bookcase. I recognized this coincidence and decided that it was time for me to read the book.

I also bought a do-it-yourself blood test kit so that I could determine my blood type. After pricking my finger and dropping my blood on a piece of paper with reagents, I determined that my blood type was O. (The next day I asked my mother about this and was told me that our entire family is O type. Moral of the story: If you want to know your blood type, and save the money on the blood test kit, just ask your mother.)

I followed the O Blood Type Diet to the letter for thirty days.

For me, this meant cutting out all dairy, wheat, pork, potatoes, corn-based products, refined sugar, peanuts, and selected fruits and vegetables. Of these foods, wheat, corn, and dairy were the only two that I was consuming regularly. I ate only free range organic meats (small quantities) and organic vegetables. It was not as difficult as it sounds and if you feel really bad, this is a very small sacrifice. Within 30 days my allergies were under control. The inhaler and drugs were no longer necessary. I was amazed and relieved by this incredible transformation.

Miraculously, my asthma was completely gone! I was breathing effortlessly and felt no symptoms whatsoever. The other by-product of my new diet was that I lost 8 pounds. I felt incredible and was really pleased with the results. This experience made me a believer in this diet and its capacity to treat all sorts of illnesses. Another appealing aspect of this diet is that it can be easily followed by a frequent traveler like me.

Growing up I was taught that allergies are a normal part of life that one just accepts and takes over-the-counter drugs to combat. In my opinion, allergies are not our "natural state;" not a normal, healthy condition. To me they are a disease that can be relieved and, in some cases, completely eliminated by simply eating natural foods. If your body is not hard at work fighting a food allergy, it will have more time and energy to devote to fighting the external allergies and bacteria that are impacting it. My own personal experience shows this to be true.

Asthma was the worst side-effect of my allergies. I discovered, during several bouts with asthma, that there are two kinds: extrinsic and intrinsic. I had a combination of the two.

"Extrinsic" asthma is caused by the antigen/antibody reaction described earlier in this chapter. Triggers can be foods, molds, and pollens. "Intrinsic" asthma is caused by emotional upset, infection, and cold air. It's sometimes referred to as "runner's asthma".

Here are the top seven food categories that I avoid[4]:

Pork	Biblically forbidden by Jews. Moslems, Hindus, Buddhists, and certain Christians also refuse this food source for centuries. I grew up eating pork. Now I generally avoid it.
Corn	All forms. In many processed foods and a staple of the Mexican diet. I love corn, but have cut way back due to allergies.
Wheat & bread	All forms, but especially refined, white flour. Replaced with sprouted Ezekiel bread. Impossible to avoid wheat entirely, but I avoid it when I can.
Potatoes	Mostly white, but especially processed potatoes like French fries. Eat occasionally.
Dairy	Milk and Cheese, especially moldy cheese like bleu cheese. Ice cream is the worst. Goat cheese is OK. Avoid most of the time.
Sugar	Especially white, refined sugar, but, sugar is sugar so it needs to be avoided, if possible. Have curtailed consumption of white sugar, but do indulge in sweets occasionally.
Peanuts, peanut butter, cashews	Staples of my childhood diet. Common allergens. I have almost eliminated peanut-based products from my diet.
Grain-fed meats	Chicken, Beef, Turkey that has been fed alot of corn should be avoided. At home I eat strictly grass fed.

4 These are foods that I found to produce allergy symptoms in me if consumed routinely.

So, you see, there are some dietary sacrifices here. Mine are lentils, potatoes, corn, peanut butter, yogurt, coffee, ice cream, and bacon. I still drink coffee and eat all of these other foods from time to time, but, not often. How do you avoid corn tacos in Mexico? I go to Mexico all of the time and can tell you that avoiding corn, a staple of their diet, is impossible. You do the best you can and eat consciously most of the time. My small sacrifice was well worth the freedom from drugs and the ability to breathe again.

Nutritional Genomics: More Scientific proof that food is a root cause of illness.

New processes developed in genetic research labs have created tests that can show your genetic profile and the foods most likely to cause disease in an individual.

One of these is the link between lectins and antigens in the Blood Type Diet causing disease, scientists have found food interactions linked to genes.

There is a particular gene called "Apo E", carried by an estimated 15% to 30% of the population, that indicates a higher risk for heart disease and diabetes. People with this gene need to avoid smoking, drinking, and the consumption of saturated fats-or die of heart disease. You may say this applies to everybody, but in fact, it applies to 100% of people with the Apo E gene. Exercise and diet, plus tee-totaling can eliminate the risk completely for Apo E gene carriers. Not fun, but this knowledge is a life saver.

There are helpful dietary recommendations for all genetic types. Get the test and find out exactly how your body reacts to certain foods. Your life may depend on it.

Genomic nutrition is further evidence that cures are an individual thing and that you should understand your blood type and in a more advanced sense, your genetics.

pH Diet—Base foods

The opposite of pH-acid is pH-alkaline.

There is a whole movement growing around the pH Diet. I first heard about the significance of the Acid/Alkaline balance 20+ years ago when I practiced the macrobiotic way of eating. Since then many books, websites, kits, and a whole slew of ways to manage pH for better health have appeared.

The basic premise is that diseases, particularly cancer, thrive in an acidic environment. The presence of life-giving oxygen is lower in an acid environment, starving our cells and making them less capable of defending themselves against intruders like viruses, bacteria, micro toxins, nano bacteria, and cancer cells. A higher mineral content is also present in high pH environments.

The acidic state is created by eating foods like refined white flour and sugar, dairy products, starches, coffee, alcohol, soda pop, hydrogenated oils, red meat, pork, some citrus fruits, and generally any heavily processed, refined food. The American junk food diet is highly acidic and generally credited with creating the higher levels of diabetes, cardiovascular disease, cancer, autoimmune diseases, and obesity found in American society today.

To reverse the acidic condition of the blood and strengthen the body, it is recommended that people consume foods that are more alkaline in nature, such as green leafy vegetables, selected grains and legumes, and drink plenty of pure water. The pH Diet calls for drinking "green drinks" like barley grass or wheat grass juice, as well as a lot of pure water and small quantities of hydrogen peroxide, which is a powerful oxygenator. I added to this, as a later stage discovery, ionized or alkaline water which is easy and very convenient to take.

Dietary supplements that neutralize acid, such as calcium and omega-3 fatty acids, are also recommended.

The pH Diet restricts all fermented foods like vinegar, wine, beer, and pickled products. (Shucks, I love these!) Most decadent food, drink, and smoking are strictly forbidden.

To test pH you urinate first thing in the morning on a piece of litmus paper. The paper changes color based on the acidity or alkalinity of your body fluid. Blue is good. Yellow is bad. The acid to alkaline scale generally runs between 3 (yellow color litmus paper) to 10.0 (dark purple litmus paper). A range between 7.0 to 7.6 is considered very good. (I actually fall below these ranges because I drink coffee and alcohol. I consciously offset my habits with alkaline foods and beverages. Nobody is perfect.)

A partial list of alkaline foods

Alkaline pH	Alkaline water, fresh spinach, broccoli, sweet potatoes, onions, lemons and limes, asparagus, blueberries, lettuce, olive oil, potato skins, tomatoes
Neutral	Tap water, butter, raw cow's milk, vegetable and nut oils
Acidic pH	Reverse osmosis water, distilled water, most bottled water, coffee, white bread, peanuts, pork, beef, wheat, cheese, pickles, pastries, shellfish, corn, rice, tomato sauce, tea, Sweet and Low, stress, worry, lack of sleep, over work, hate

Note: Partial list from my experience, the pH Miracle, and other sources.[5]

---

5   *Young, Robert O. PhD and Young, Shelly Redford. The pH Miracle. Warner Books New York, NY. 2002.pp 79–80 Note: I discovered the Alkaline dietary guidelines with the mac¬robiotic diet but attained a better understanding reading this book. I am not giving the pH diet detailed coverage because there are so many books and websites that cover this topic. In nutrition circles, this is a well known concept.*

My Experience

I have never followed the pH Diet strictly, but do incorporate some of its principles into my diet and periodically test my pH level. The biggest step undertaken to "get pH" was the acquisition of a water ionizer (See Chapter 18). This is a huge, helpful shortcut to removing a lot of acid from your body.

Because of the coffee and alcohol I drink and the red meat that I eat, my body fluids are generally on the acidic side of the scale. Even though I do not go overboard, the litmus test results are typically between 6.6 to 6.8, which aren't bad, but are below the desired 7.0+ reading. When cutting back on acidic foods, it is quickly reflected in the pH test, which rises above 7.0. Drinking a few quarts a day of alkaline water also helps.

I have introduced a number of people to the pH Diet and most find it way too restrictive to their tastes. It is essentially a vegan diet with some provisions for fish. But if you are sick, this is a healing diet to the max. Do it. It is much better than being in the hospital.

What I tell people is "desperate times require desperate measures", so if you want to get better, reduce the acid in your body by any means possible. This will save you a lot of unnecessary misery.

If you eat the typical American diet, you will not like this one, but it will make you healthy. If I were to be diagnosed with cancer I would follow the pH Diet to the letter and remain confident that it would help me. There is no doubt in my mind that if you oxygenate and purify your blood, you are well equipped to battle cancer without killing yourself in the process with chemotherapy. This goes for any disease, for that matter. It has been written that cancer cannot survive in an alkaline environment. It needs an acid, anaerobic (oxygen-starved) environment to grow and multiply. These facts are well documented in books and research.

I highly recommend this diet to anyone who is sick or is looking for a way to completely cleanse their body and get into top physical condition. You need self-discipline and access to pH Diet foods and supplements to succeed.

> Green drinks, alfalfa tablets, seas veggies, lemon water, water, kukicha tea with umeboeshi plum, wheat grass juice, and most importantly ionized water are important alkalizing foods.

Mixing Foods: Here's a useful health tip I bet you'll never follow (like me)

> The digestion of protein, starch and sugar requires different digestive processes. Combining more than one type of these foods prevents some of the food from digesting. This undigested food gets trapped in your intestinal tract and rots, causing all sorts of unpleasantries. The Western diet, and many others, is full of poor food combinations that should be avoided, if you want optimum digestion.
>
> - Do not mix proteins. (Example: Surf (lobster) and turf (beef), bacon and beef)
> - Do not mix dairy products. (Example: Cheese with a glass of milk)
> - Do not mix proteins and most starches. (Example: Meat and potatoes, fish and chips)
> - Do not combine sugar and starch. (Example: Apple pie)
> - Do not combine sugar and protein. (Example: Sugar glazed pork ribs)

Sounds like a lot of fun doesn't it? This is a tough set of guidelines for most people to follow. All cuisines combine proteins, starches, and sugars. It is part of the fun of eating.

I strictly follow these guidelines only when I am sick, which is infrequently. I am totally conscious of these combinations and usually avoid mixing foods, when possible. For example, I rarely eat potatoes with meat or fish like most people because of the starch/protein interaction. Animal protein is something that you want fully digested. Undigested meat can cause a lot of problems. Because my diet is roughly 75% vegetables and 25% animal protein, I only have to think about this mixing issue 25% of the time, so I generally don't worry about it. But, if I feel lousy, I follow these guidelines to a "T". Try it. You may feel better.

The Glycemic Index (GI)

The Glycemic Index is a measure that ranks carbohydrate-rich foods by how they raise blood glucose levels compared to pure glucose or white bread. When you eat foods that contain sugar (glucose), your blood glucose level rises. The speed that the food is able to increase your blood glucose level is called the "glycemic response" which is impacted by the quantity of food that you eat and how the food is actually prepared. Foods that raise your blood glucose levels quickly have a high glucose index rating.

I am not a biochemist or doctor so I will not delve into the details, but will give it to you in the simplistic way that I understand it.

Here is another very useful quick guide for your health that is no fun at all for us junk food eaters and drinkers, but it may save your life. You'll notice a not coincidental relationship between high glycemic foods and high pH acidity. There is a correlation between all of this healing stuff.

---

6 Dispenza, Joseph. *Live Better Longer. The Parcels Center 7—Step Plan for Health and Longevity.* Lincoln, NE : iUniverse.com, Inc. 1997, 2000. Pp 57–59

Managing the Glycemic Response: Good Carbs versus Bad Carbs

The GI is at the core of just about every major, effective diet and, if understood and practiced as a meal planning tool with regularity, it will help you to regulate blood sugar (blood glucose level), enhance weight loss, improve thinking, reduce cholesterol, improve your mood, and reduce the effects of most other debilitating diseases. Children with learning disabilities and behavior issues can gain huge benefits by reducing their sugar intake and managing the Glycemic Index of their diet.

In my studies, the common theme throughout most of the legitimate diets and health regimens is the proper management of sugar consumption. Consuming good carbs (low glycemic foods) versus bad carbs (high glycemic foods) is a critical health factor. SUGAR KILLS! Low glycemic foods should be consumed in conjunction with medium glycemic foods for maximum health.

Many diabetics understand and follow the Glycemic Index since insulin levels are critical to their health. The same concerns that diabetics have for glucose levels should be shared by non-diabetics, as we are all susceptible to getting type 2 diabetes, if we do not watch our consumption of bad carbs over the long-haul.

Refined sugar, refined flour, and all foods derived from these sources, are high Glycemic Index foods and highly acidic. These foods should be minimized or avoided to promote good health.

Enjoy your sweets by eating sugars that slowly raise your glucose levels like barley malt or rice syrup, if possible.

When you eat foods that contain sugar (glucose) your blood glucose level raises. The speed that the food is able to increase your blood glucose level is called the "glycemic response" which is impacted by the quantity of food that you eat and how the food is actually prepared. Foods that raise your blood glucose levels quickly have a high glucose index rating.

Here is a summary chart of Low, Medium, and High glycemic foods. Perform a web search on the Glycemic Index[1] to locate the entire GI food list.

Low Glycemic Foods Scale (55 or less) "Good Carbs"

Chick peas (humus)	Whole oats
Oat bran	Sweet potatoes
Soy milk	Apples
Plain yogurt	Baked beans
Green veggies	

Medium Glycemic Index foods (56–69) "OK Carbs"

Banana	Basmati rice
Raisins	Whole wheat bread
Popcorn	New potatoes
Brown rice	

High Glycemic Foods (69++) "Bad Carbs"

White Table sugar (sucrose)	Corn Flakes™
Instant mashed potatoes	Soda Crackers
Baked white potatoes	White bagels
High fructose corn syrup (sweetener used in most soda pop)	White flour
Rice Krispies™	French fries
Cheerios™	Ice Cream

1   Glycemic Index—website—Canadian Diabetic Association. http://www.diabetes.ca/

You get the drift. This should be common sense...fast food, junk food, and all the other highly processed stuff consumed in massive quantities by Americans is generally high GI and should be considered a treat instead of a daily diet. When carbs are refined they are absorbed into the body faster causing negative results.

Complex carbs are "time released" causing a gradual increase in blood glucose. It's like the difference between mainlining sugar and taking a time-release capsule that releases it into your system gradually.

For some, changing these habits will not happen. For others, a gradual weaning process will take place, health will be restored, and the old way of high GI eating will become a distant memory. We need as many people as possible to accept the low GI way of eating as our healthcare system cannot keep up with all the sickness and disease caused by high GI foods in this country. Our junk food diet is spreading around the world, making once healthy people sick.

Note: There are some subtleties in the GI that you need to be aware of. For example, a Snickers bar is lower on the GI than a baked potato. Is the Snickers bar better? No. White rice is only 3 points higher than brown rice. White rice is almost as good? Incorrect. Brown rice has more nutrients and fiber than white rice which has been bleached and stripped of most nutritional value. Some common sense needs to be applied when using the GI guide.

My Experience

I grew up on sugar and have the cavity fillings in my teeth to prove it. Candy and soda pop were staples of my diet. They were for sale in my elementary school, candy stores on the way home from school, in movie theaters, at sporting events, just about everywhere I went. I was a little sugar junkie. So were 80% of the children with whom I associated. You wouldn't know it looking at me now, but I was built on sugar, lots of sugar. This is the foundation of the American fast food diet and the root of all of the major illnesses we are experiencing today. It is one of the reasons that I sometimes overcompensate in the area of nutrition as an adult. I have a lot of youthful mistakes to make up for!

Not until my high school years did I naturally begin weaning myself off of sugar. My motivation? Girls! I loved girls and wanted to attract them. I quickly learned the sugar/zit/pimple (skin blemish) connection and was vain enough to want as few zits as possible to make myself attractive to the opposite sex. So I cut way, way back on my sugar intake and noticed almost immediately that my complexion cleared up. This is one of the two helpful applications of vanity that I have discovered in my life. There are only two.

My gratitude for all life's lessons

I thank pimples for curbing my voracious appetite for sugar. It's a fact. My burning desire to expel every blemish from my teenage body was the entryway to a higher consciousness diet. I did not do this because it was good for me; I did it for self love and vanity. Whatever works! This worked for me.

As I stopped eating candy and cut way back on sugar, my dietary preferences naturally changed from eating junk to eating fresh vegetables, fruits, whole grains, and protein-rich foods. Unknowingly, I was naturally detoxifying my body. In return, my body signaled back what it needed to replenish the vitamins and minerals that I had depleted during years of sugar abuse.

Highly processed carbs, like instant mashed potatoes, instant rice, instant oatmeal, instant drinks, most breakfast cereals, soda pop, refined sugar, and refined flour-based products, were slowly moving out of my diet.

The other healthy exercise in vanity (Number 2) that I picked up in puberty was weight lifting. My older brother, Howard, was an avid weightlifter in college so I was well aware of the benefits of this training. I found his old rusting set of weights in the basement, sprayed them with Rustoleum and began lifting four to five times a week. I was 14 years old when this started. This was another activity whose sole purpose was for attracting girls. It worked!

Teenagers, here's a tip you won't want to miss!

> **Note to Teen Girls and Boys: Get more dates!** Lose your zits and excess fat. Stop eating sugar and French fries. It will get rid of your excess fat and zits. Lift weights. Toned bodies get the attention of the opposite sex. Don't do either of these because I say so, do it so you will attract the opposite sex. You will go out on more dates. I guarantee it! This works ... I know it does.

At 14 years of age I obviously did not know it, but exercise has a huge impact on how glucose is burned in the body with training and exercise of any kind. Your muscles burn glucose as energy, depleting the supply in your body and making good use of blood glucose. This is why sports drinks contain so much glucose. They are glucose replacement therapy. The recommended use of them is only after extreme physical exertion where an athlete has perspired and lost a lot of body water. These drinks have been mistaken for nutritional beverage-, which they are not. They are horrible for you unless you are burning lots of calories and glucose.

So it sounds like the Glycemic Index takes all of the fun out of eating and life doesn't it? It will if you become a GI fanatic. However, the value of the GI is to become aware of what you are doing and make the best food choice the majority of the time.

Everything in moderation including moderation!

I do not follow the GI to a "T" because I like too many different foods and like to indulge myself (in moderation) every so often. However, I am aware of the GI of what I am eating and the physical consequences that come with the consumption of these foods. So, when I get a sugar rush and then tired an hour later, I know exactly why that happened. If I get hyper, I know that it was the soda I drank or the candy I ate. Since I don't like feeling hyper, I rarely drink soda or eat candy. Applied knowledge is power. As stated in the beginning, we all have choices. You can choose to feel good or bad and in many cases it's the food you eat making you feel that way.

Over consumption of high GI foods can lead to diabetes, obesity, cancer, heart disease, and many other debilitating diseases.
Eat good carbs, avoid bad carbs, drink pure water, exercise, and you can probably skip the rest of this book. Although, of course, I wouldn't recommend the last option!

If you insist on eating crap, at least increase your water intake and take a vegetable supplement, such as alfalfa or sea vegetable tablets.
Note to men and women over 40. Just like the teenagers getting rid of pimples, you'll get rid of that dumpy posterior and potbelly by following the Glycemic Index and eliminating high Glycemic Index foods. The results will be miraculous! The weight will drop, your energy will increase, and your overall health will improve.

"The table kills more people than war does."
— Catalan Proverb

Chapter 4
Vitamins & Supplements

Personally, I have taken vitamins since I was a child and continue to do so today, with some guidelines provided by a competent nutritionist. Nutrition is an individual thing like all healing. You need different vitamins and minerals at different times in your life. There are a few global recommendations that can be made for everyone, but it's mostly an individual thing. That is why nutritionists have a job.

Here's the truth according to me: If you have access to, and can eat locally grown, natural, organic vegetables, fruits, grains, and meats, you require a minimal amount of vitamin and mineral supplementation. All you need is contained in the fresh healthy food that you eat. However, if you are a vegetarian, you'll probably need supplementation to make up for the vitamins you're missing from animal protein, such as vitamin B12 and Coenzyme Q10.

In Austin we are blessed with a 12-month growing season and four farmers' markets within a 30 minute drive of my house that support organic or chemical-free farming. They call this "slow food." (This is food raised the old-fashioned way before the industrialization of farming and mass production. There are no pesticides or chemical fertilizers, antibiotics and growth hormones used.) Local food is not shipped long distances nor stored for any length of time so it retains its nutritional value. Also, since it is local, it helps you eat according to the season and consume food that is part of your local environment, which is in keeping with macrobiotics and other natural schools of living.

I am a big fan of this way of eating and a dedicated practitioner. Come over to my house on any given weekend and I will knock your socks off with locally grown, minimally processed, fresh, well-cooked or raw foods, while we drink some good beer or wine and maybe enjoy a good cigar.

This abundance of locally grown, natural foods is a blessing that most people in America do not have. When I travel outside of Austin, which is frequently, I take vitamin and mineral supplements. The food served in most restaurants is commercially grown and missing a lot of its nutrients because of the way it was grown, transported, stored, and processed.

There are three general categories of vitamin production: synthetic, extracts, and natural. Synthetic vitamins, as the name suggests, are man-made in a test tube with inorganic substances not easily absorbed by the body and can have harmful side effects. Extracts are not much better than synthetics in that they typically consist of 10% or less natural ingredients, contain very few enzymes, have harsh fillers, and use low quality raw materials. Natural vitamins use natural sources for their ingredients, such as fruits and vegetables, have natural enzymes, and are easily absorbed by the body.

You are better off not taking any vitamins if they are synthetic or as extracts as they are toxic. You might as well chew on plastic. Get naturally derived vitamins or skip them all together.

Before you start taking supplements, you should consult a qualified nutritionist to pinpoint exactly what it is that your body needs. The Asyra 3 bio-energetic health screening system, discussed in Chapter 11, is a great way to find this out.

My Experience

My personal Vitamins, Minerals, and Supplements[2]

Vitamin/Mineral	Description/Benefit	Sources
Magnesium*	Involved in 300+ enzyme reactions. Calms nerves, helps assimilate calcium, and enhances cardiovascular function. Take immediately after a heart attack for recovery assistance. According to Norman Shealy, MD, PhD, 90% of Americans suffer from a magnesium deficiency. This supplement is essential for me.	Broccoli, kale, spinach, almonds, raisins
Calcium*	The most abundant mineral in the body. Found in bones, teeth, and bodily fluids. Alkaline. Helps reduce acid state.	Supplements, soy milk, green leafy vegetables
Potassium	Electrolyte. The athlete's friend. Controls fluid movement into and out of tissues and cells.	Artichokes, kale, sweet potatoes, spinach
Omega-3 and omega-6 fatty acids*	Present in human cells (brain, nerve), adrenal glands, and hasr anti-clotting properties. Good for cardiovascular function.	Cold water fish oils, like salmon, halibut, cod. Flaxseed and soybean oils

2   Shaklee Corporation—"What Will Shaklee Supplements Do?" A data sheet from the Shaklee Nutrition Resource Center. Also based on my 20+ years of supplementation.

Vitamins & Supplements

Vitamin/Mineral	Description/Benefit	Sources
Vitamin C*	Humans are the only animal that cannot produce this. "Old Faithful" has a beneficial effect in every bodily function, particularly as an antioxidant.	Parsley, kale, collard greens, strawberries, broccoli, French sorrel
CoQ 10	Aids in protecting cells from free radical damage. Produces energy in all cells of the body. Not readily available in most foods. Good for the heart.	Supplements, organic bison or beef liver; organ meats
Sodium (salt)	Most common trace mineral and condiment.	Evaporated sea water
Selenium	Mineral antioxidant. Helps with heart function and free radical protection.	Bison meat, carrots, artichokes, asparagus, broccoli (no supplements)
Zinc	Immune system protection. Used as cold remedy. Reproductive aid. Increases sperm count.	Seafood, whole grains, organic meat
Iron	Transports oxygen throughout the body via red blood cells. Body's basic building block.	Chicken, fish, meat, nuts, whole grains, broccoli

Vitamin/Mineral	Description/Benefit	Sources
Vitamin D	The "sunshine drug." Vitamin D is produced in the kidneys and converted into the hormone calcitrol. Calcitrol helps assimilate calcium into the body. Thought to have significant cancer fighting properties.	Sunshine at least 30+ minutes 5 times a week. Get your sunshine, but don't burn. Vitamin supplements in small doses, if sunshine is in short supply.
Beta-carotene Vitamin A	Beta-carotene is the yellow, orange, and red pigment found in many vegetables. It is converted into vitamin A by the body. Antioxidant and free radical scavenger that promotes healing in many areas. Helps with eyesight and vision.	Sweet potatoes, carrots, peppers, cucumbers, squash, broccoli, green leafy vegetables. Abundant in fruits and vegetables.
Vitamin B6	Metabolism of amino acids and proteins. Helps with the production of hemoglobin in the blood and the function of neurotransmitters. A deficiency adversely affects your mood and sleep. "Brain food."	Organ meats, meat, potato skins, brewer's yeast, wheat germ, bananas, beans
Vitamin B12	Supports growth of cells, and red blood cell production.	Eggs, meat, milk, cheese

Vitamins & Supplements

Vitamin/Mineral	Description/Benefit	Sources
Probiotics*	Lactobacillus acidophilus, Lactobacillus bulgaricus, Lactobacillus casel, Streptococcus thermophilus, Bifidobacterium longum, etc. "Friendly" bacteria for the intestinal flora. This is "good bacteria" that fights bad bacteria when it enters your body. They inhibit the growth of yeast and other disease-causing bacteria. I use them daily.	Probiotic supplements with at least 1 billion live organisms per gram. Cultured yogurt or kifir contain probiotics supplements are best. These are my number one supplement. I use PRO EM•1® Daily Probotic Cleanse
Digestive enzymes*	Assists food digestion, particularly animal protein, insuring better absorption of vitamins and minerals.	Bromelain, an enzyme found in fresh papaya and pineapple. Capsules containing a mixture of digestive enzymes.
Trace minerals	Germanium, iodine, zinc, palladium, molybdenum, indium and anything that can be found in sea water. Excellent for removing heavy metals from the body. Thyroid health. Alkaline characteristics…	Sea vegetables (dulse, wakame, kombu, kelp)
Protein Amino acids	Basic building blocks of life. Muscle nutrition.	Soybean curd and soy tempeh. Grass-fed bison, beef, chicken.

Rich Remedies

Vitamin/Mineral	Description/Benefit	Sources
Vitamin E	Alpha Tocopheral, a powerful antioxidant known to fight free radical damage. Beneficial effects in cardiovascular health and fighting certain types of cancer. Said to work best in combination with beta-carotene, selenium, and vitamin C.	Soybeans, nuts, green leafy vegetables
Vitamin K	Aids in blood clotting.	Eggs
Kukicha Tea Umeboeshi Plum	Kukicha tea, made from the twigs of tea plants, is alkaline in nature and contains iron and other minerals. Umeboeshi plum is a pickled Japanese plum having alkaline properties. Macrobiotic beverage. Lowers acidity, aids digestion, has anti-parasitic effects.	Tea plant, Japanese umeboeshi plums
Garlic	Concentrated garlic extract provides high doses of acillin (active ingredient in garlic), along with having anti-parasitic and antibacterial properties. Lowers cholesterol. Cleanses blood.	Garlic cloves

Taken daily, your supplements will be different than mine based on the recommendations of your healing coach.

Vitamins & Supplements

Comments about the Vitamin, Mineral, and Supplement Chart

The vitamins and supplements above are my personal preference. You will need to find the combination that works for you and your present state of wellness.

Many people in the United States, even over-weight people, suffer from some type of malnutrition because the fast food and junk food they consume contains "empty" calories. Their excess weight is due to a lack of good nutrition, not an excess of nutrition as one would imagine. An aid to weight loss and wellness should include the use of vitamins and supplements, as appropriate and under the guidance of a nutritionist, as well as diet modification. Not many people eat as conscientiously as I do, so more vitamins and minerals may be appropriate.

A good wide spectrum multivitamin is the easiest way to cover the bases. Make sure though that the supplement is naturally derived from vegetables and fruits and has more than the recommended daily allowance (RDA) of key nutrients. (Note that you don't see a multivitamin on my list. This is because I have a nutritionist-guided dietary program and an awareness of what I need.) Most people I know require a multivitamin, in addition to other supplements, in order to get all of the nutrition they need. I do occasionally take a multivitamin, but it is based on nutritional recommendations from a professional healing coach.

If you are taking medication, always check for counter-interactions between the medicine and the supplement. Some counteract each other and, in rare cases, are actually toxic in combination, so it is a good idea to check with your physician before taking any form of supplement.

Examples:
- Vitamin E should not be taken while on a blood clotting medication. Vitamin E has natural blood anticoagulation (thinning) properties that will actually interact negatively

with blood clotting medications.

- Acidophilus binds with antibiotics so it is good to take them before and after a course of antibiotics but not during antibiotic treatment. I have gotten conflicting opinions on this one, but I believe for me they work best before and after. Check with your healing coach.

- The supplements that I use frequently fit my needs best (magnesium, omega-3, and vitamin C) have anti-inflammatory properties that are good for managing my allergies.

Digestive Enzymes and Probiotics

These two became a part of my regimen uponI learning of their importance during cleansing therapies. Proper "bowel care" is essential to your health. Many diseases (70% +) originate in your bowel (in addition to your mind) and can be best addressed there. Proper digestion, especially of animal products, is aided by digestive enzymes which help with the assimilation and eventual elimination of food. Probiotics maintain healthful bacteria, keeping molds and other micro toxins in check. There is a battle going on between "good bacteria and "bad bacteria" all the time. Populating your digestive tract with probiotics gives you an advantage in fighting off bacteria that cause sickness. This is a very, very important supplement. Most diseases start in the gut. Proper gut health is paramount.

Before taking any supplements, you should have a blood analysis and urine analysis or, as I have discovered, a Bio-Energetic Health Screening. Otherwise you're guessing. A trained professional can determine some of the telltale symptoms of a mineral or vitamin deficiency by just listening to a patient's health issues; like they do on radio health talk shows. This takes years of clinical experience and is still, to some degree, guess work. If you really want to know what you need, get tested. Bio-Energetic Health

Screening is now my preferred method. Informed nutrition is good nutrition and it will save you money in the long run.

Cleansing

No supplements for cleansing are listied in the matrix because it's not supplementation in that sense, but it does help with overall nutrition. I cleanse 2 to 3 times a year depending on how I feel. There are a bunch of easy to use cleansing supplements available that make this process trouble-free and effective. I highly recommend that you do something to "clean out the basement." You do it for your house, septic system, and car's engine so why wouldn't you do it for your body? I know why. It's gross; disgusting to some. Just do it. Getting your diaper and bedpan changed as an adult in a hospital is worse. This process is discussed further in Chapter 6, Internal Cleansing.

The medical lobby has been trying to regulate the sale of vitamins and supplement sales for years through Codex Alimentarus and other subterfuge methods. They want you to have a prescription for supplements just like you have for their drugs, leading me to conclude that supplements are good for you and do play a role in preventing disease. Healthy people reduce the need for drugs and hospitalization.

Lipid Exchange and Phosphatidyl Choline (PC) Are Truly Amazing!! The Ultimate Life-Giving Turbo-Charged Omega Fatty Acids!

I know! I keep saying that this XYZ natural cure is miraculous, so, when I say it again, you'll probably disregard my enthusiasm as more puffery. But don't do that here.

I'm convinced that Phosphatidylcholine (PC) and the therapies developed at the Haverford Wellness Center located in Pennsylvania are truly miraculous. People travel thousands of miles to receive these breakthrough, life-changing natural therapies for many chronic diseases. They are all natural and work!

PC has been clinically proven to dramatically improve outcomes for patients with disorders such as Alzheimer's, ALS, Lyme Disease, Parkinson's, MS, Fibromyalgia, Chronic Fatigue Syndrome, Autism, seizures, Hepatitis C, environmental toxins, cardiovascular disease, and more.[1]

The body's cell membranes are where life begins and ends. By feeding and strengthening the cell membranes you extend life. For more information see the section on colon hydrotherapy in Chapter 6. I discuss the clinical experience of Alex Carrel, MD, a Nobel Prize winning physician. He kept chicken embryos alive for 29 years by keeping the fluid around the cell membrane toxin free. The membrane is the most important part of the cell.

Another example of extending cell life comes from Dr. Ed Kane, PhD and his wife Dr. Patricia Kane, PhD, who have backgrounds in nutrition and biochemistry. They are the top researchers in PC today and involved in the clinical trials and research on PC at the Haverford Wellness Center.

A 1985 study done at Hebrew University by Yechtel and Barenholtz highlighted the relationship between aging, disease, and the role of Phosphatidylcholine in slowing these processes. Using rat heart cells they demonstrated the ability of PC to fully rejuvenate cells that were almost dead, providing evidence of the importance of PC at the cellular level. More detailed information can be found at Yechiel E., Barenholz Y.,J.Biol Chem 1985 Aug 5, 260 (16):9123.

> "PC directly up-regulates the fluidity of the cell membrane, improving its health which is essential for all metabolism including neural transmission. Poor Neural response is degraded in all the neurological disorders and is directly improved with PC therapy. Raising PC levels plays an

---

[1] *Haverford Wellness Center website www.haverfordwellness.com/about*

> important role in improving memory and recall, and has clinically shown to improve the flow of information of all the senses and most significantly the eyesight. PC given either orally or intravenously helps restore the proper integrity of the cell membrane thereby restoring proper function of organ systems, especially the liver, the gut, the brain, immune system, heart, and hormonal system which ultimately improves the total health of the individual."[2]

This is essentially an anti-aging formula that trickles down to the cellular level. The "secret sauce" here is the essential omega-6 and omega-3 fatty acids in an optimized ratio of 4:1 which is the exact proportion that makes up 70% of a cell membrane, and is exactly the amount your cells need in order to regenerate. This is a "super nutrient" that helps nature at the cellular level repair itself. PC resonates with your cells.

My Experience

PC is a very recent discovery for me, courtesy of my naturopath, Meridian Grace, ND. (My verdict on PC's effectiveness won't be in by the time this book is published.) I am currently on a 9-month program designed by Dr. Patricia Kane that is said to be effective against those neurotoxins that are the root cause of disease and aging.

My *intention* is to proactively remove the majority of the neurotoxins from my body in order to reduce the probability of my getting a chronic disease. If successful, I believe that this therapy, more than anything else in my medicine bag, will shave 10 years of aging off my body and significantly improve my quality of life.

---

2   Yechiel E, Barenholzy.,J.Biol Chem 1985 Aug 5, 260 (16) :9123. Haverford Wellness Center, BodyBio Bulletin, part number 902.2, www.bodybio.com

I'm convinced, from what I have read, is that PC will work for me. My expected outcomes: reducing my cholesterol level from its present level of 236 to below 220, reduction of ten (10) years in physical aging of my body, clearer thoughts, better eyesight, and more energy. Who knows? I'll let you know. Stay tuned.

I refer you to BodyBio Bulletin, part number 902.2 from www.bodybio.com. This is an eight page brochure that will tell you everything you need to know about PC and includes short case studies of successful treatments of **Parkinson's, ALS, Alzheimer's, MS, and Autism**. Truly Amazing!

NutriFeron®

Pumpkin seed extract, safflower extract, Asian plantago seed extract, and Japanese honeysuckle flower extract…NutriFeron®… an amazing natural immune system booster.[3] Always on the lookout for cool stuff, I found this unique remedy quite by accident.

I called Shaklee Corporation and they directed me to the company's home page. There I found a small section on NutriFeron®, their exclusive patented plant-based version of Interferon. It fascinated me that me that a natural form of this miracle drug was available in pill form for less than fifty bucks a bottle. (The man-made version is off the charts expensive.) NutriFeron® was discovered by Yashuiko Kojima, PhD, one of the original researchers who developed Interferon in the 1950s. It took him forty years of research, studying of Chinese medicinal herbs and experimenting with over 200 botanicals, to find a combination that would help the human body naturally manufacture its own Interferon.

Interferon is one of a group of proteins called "cytokines", which act as chemical messengers, triggering immune responses in your body. They send a signal to the cells that an invading pathogen (bacteria, virus, or toxin) is in your blood and calls the

---

[3] Shaklee Corporation have the exclusive rights to NutriFeron® See www.shaklee.com/rich, NutriFeron®

[4] Center for Immune Research, Clinical Abstracts, http://www.naturalinterferon.com/clinical.html Pages 1–4 and see www.shaklee.net/rich, NutriFeron®.

surrounding cells into action. It "interferes" with how foreign cells, like cancers, grow and multiply. To put it more simply, Interferon is like the worker bee that signals to the other worker bees that an invader is in the hive and instructs them to attack. And attack they do, with a vengeance! Interferon works the same way in your body and is, perhaps, best known as an antiviral agent in the treatment of HIV/AIDS, rabies, herpes, and hepatitis C. The fancy term for this immune system response is *"the complement destruction cascade."* (I love this term! Sounds like a play out of the Philadelphia Eagles' playbook.)4Your body is at work 24 hours a day, 7 days a week. When this process degrades, you are more susceptible to viruses, cancer, and other diseases. Compromised, they don't act with the same gusto as when they are at full strength.

Influenza, a form of virus, can be treated with Interferon, but the side effects, dizziness, headache, depression, and exhaustion, may be worse than the flu itself, so it is not prescribed for this purpose.

A virus is a sub-microscopic particle that can infect the cells of a biological organism. Viruses can only reproduce by infecting a host cell, using its life energy for its own growth and nourishment.. They cannot reproduce on their own like bacteria. Also, viruses are generally not affected by antibiotics like bacteria. Your immune system is constantly battling these viruses with its own naturally produced Interferon.

Stress, sleep deprivation, pollution, poor diet, and physical exertion can weaken the immune system and make it more susceptible to disease.

My Experience

It's hard to know exactly what impact NutriFeron® has had on my immune system since I started taking it. I have successfully beaten most allergies through diet and cleansing, so adding this to the mix has thus so far been inconclusive. My allergy symptoms only emerge these days when I break my diet by eating foods that trigger an immune response, such as dairy.

The proof that there is some benefit for NutriFeron® use is probably best reflected in the clinical trials (available from Shaklee Corporation) that have been performed using it.:

- A three month study was conducted at Kanazawa University Hospital in Ishikawa, Japan, on patients with chronic hepatitis C. A reduction in depression, abdominal bloating, nausea, and vomiting occurred in patients who were taking 1 gram per day of NutriFeron.

- Three controlled trials, on 113 subjects with nasal allergies or hay fever, were conducted by researchers in Japan between 1998 and 2000. Subjects reported a reduction in sneezing, nasal discharge, teary eyes, nasal blockage, and other common hay fever symptoms.

- In a trial at Yamanashi Medical University, Japan, subjects were shown to have significant increases in blood gamma Interferon levels within 4 weeks of use, illustrating how NutriFeron® aids the body in the natural production of this immune system boosting chemical.

The clinical studies also found that there were benefits to menopausal women and those experiencing discomfort from Premenstrual Symptom (PMS). For details see the clinical trials at Center for Immune Research (http://www.naturalinterferon.com).[5]

Note: As with everything else in this book, I recommend consulting your physician before taking any vitamin or herbal supplement.

Vivix™ - Incredible Healing Tonic

As this book is going to print, I received a product notice from Shaklee Corporation announcing a revolutionary new patented anti- aging

Vitamins & Supplements

tonic called Vivix™. Incredible healing products keep surfacing as I'm trying to finish Rich Remedies, Volume 1. Vivix™ is really cool based on my preliminary review of the Shaklee information, so I'm including it here. This is the only healing remedy in this book that I have not tried on myself, since it is brand new. I will be trying it out as soon as the product starts shipping. You can learn more about Vivix at my website www.richremedies.com. Nutrition Code :Richremedies

Vivix™ contains massive amounts of resveratral, a compound found in red wine that has been linked to anti aging. Dr. David Sinclair, associate professor of pathology at Harvard University Medical School, has isolated genetic proteins at the cellular level that cause aging. He discovered that resveratrol can slow down the aging process by acting on these genes that are "longevity regulators." These genes, if controlled, will slow down the aging process according to Dr. Sinclair and many other clinical studies. The studies were performed on lab rats and mice, but evidence suggests that the aging proteins exist across a wide variety of organism and that resveratral will be effective in humans.

Shaklee Corporation has performed extensive research and optimized the resveratral manufacturing process to produce the compound in its purest, most concentrated form with additional polyphenols. This is considered their greatest nutritional discovery. During this project they also discovered a grape variety called vitis rotondifolia that contains higher concentrations of resveratrol than other varieties. Then they perfected an extraction process that maximizes the quantity and quality of the resveratral compound that goes into their Vivix™ tonic.

My premise that your best source of nutrition is locally grown, organic produce needs a small asterisk in the case of Vivix™. This is because, according to Shaklee, you would need to drink 3,000 glasses of red wine in one month to get the quantity of resveratrol

---

5 Center for Immune Research, Clinical Abstracts, httep://www.naturalinterferon.com/ clinical html pages 1–4. All references to the clinical tests for NutriFeron®

you need to slow down the aging process. One teaspoon of Vivix™ is equivalent to 100 glasses of red wine. So even if you are a two fisted red wine drinker (I know a few), it is not possible to get all the quantity of resveratral you need to slow down aging. Plus, your liver and kidneys will give out drinking all that red wine. So Vivix™ is the way you can get adequate quantities of resveratral and polyphenols to slow the aging process.

In my next book, *Rich Remedies, Volume 2*, I will share my experience with Vivix™ and provide more information than time permits at present.

These statements have not been evaluated by the Food and Drug Administration. This product is not intended to diagnose, treat, cure, or prevent disease.

Chapter 5
Herbs

Herbs have been used for centuries to heal all matter of illnesses. They are nature's pharmaceutical, along with natural foods. My introduction to healing herbs came during my sophomore year at Widener College. Since then I have grown many herbs and use them daily in food preparation.

The main reason herbs have fallen from favor as part of our daily, natural medicine, is the practice of allopathic medicine, the convenience of over-the-counter drugs, and a lack of mass media attention regarding their healing benefits. In our fast food society and era of instant gratification, highly marketed designer drugs are more convenient than herbs. Also, there are so few physicians who understand the healing properties of herbs. Herbs are not advertised or sexy. It's a lot easier to swallow a few pills than to use herbs. We are an instant gratification society. This includes me. Herbs I use regularly (weekly)[6].

Herb	Healing effects*
Garlic	Active ingredient: Acillin. Properties: Antibacterial, antifungal, blood thinning, antioxidant. Said to: Reduce cholesterol and arte¬rial plaque, and strengthen heart.
Ginger	Properties: Anti inflammatory. Used to: Treat nausea, vomiting and motion sickness and as a digestive aid.
Parsley	High in vitamin C, iron, potassium, and calcium. Properties: Used to treat: urinary infections, bad breath, and lost libido in women. (Buy it by the bushel basket guys!)

Herb	Healing effects*
Basil	Properties: Antiviral; used in folk medicine to get rid of warts; phytochemicals said to remove plaque from teeth.
Rosemary	"Herb of remembrance." Uses: Helps with blood circulation, particularly to the brain, Alzheimer's, arthritis, diabetes, indigestion, and blood pressure.
Thyme	Uses: Treatment of breathing problems, such as asthma, coughs, and bronchitis (said to be treated by doses of thyme syrup, as prescribed by a physician); also said to kill certain worms.
Cayenne	Active ingredient: Capsaicin (the phytochemical that produces the heat in peppers, such as cayenne). Uses: Anti-inflammatory, blood thinner, blood circulation, cholesterol reduction, anti-bacterial, pain reliever. Also provides a "cooling effect" in hot weather.
Onion/Shallot	Active ingredient: Quercetin, a bioflavonoid found in onion skin. Uses: anti-inflammatory. Good for treating allergies and respiratory ailments, colds, diabetes, high blood pressure and inflamed bowels.
Spearmint	Uses: Treatment of indigestion, stomach ache, bad breath, and colds.
Black Pepper	Active ingredient: peperine. Uses: Digestive aid, constipation, and said to help the body assimilate certain vitamins during the digestive process.
Oregano	Uses: Anti-microbial, antibacterial, and antifungal agent, and antiparasitic.
Chamomile	Anti-inflammatory, antibacterial, relaxes nerves, and calms the stomach.

Most of these herbs have been used by me for years and in some cases grown in my herb garden.

Note: As pharmaceuticals, healing herbs should be used only after a proper diagnosis has been made by a naturopathic doctor. The healing effects noted here are based on my personal use and research. A good resource is *The Green Pharmacy Herbal Handbook* by James A. Duke, PhD.[7]

The way I get my weekly herbs is through a healing salad dressing that I developed over a year of experimenting. You can get the complete recipe for this amazing herb dressing by going to my website www.richremedies.com.

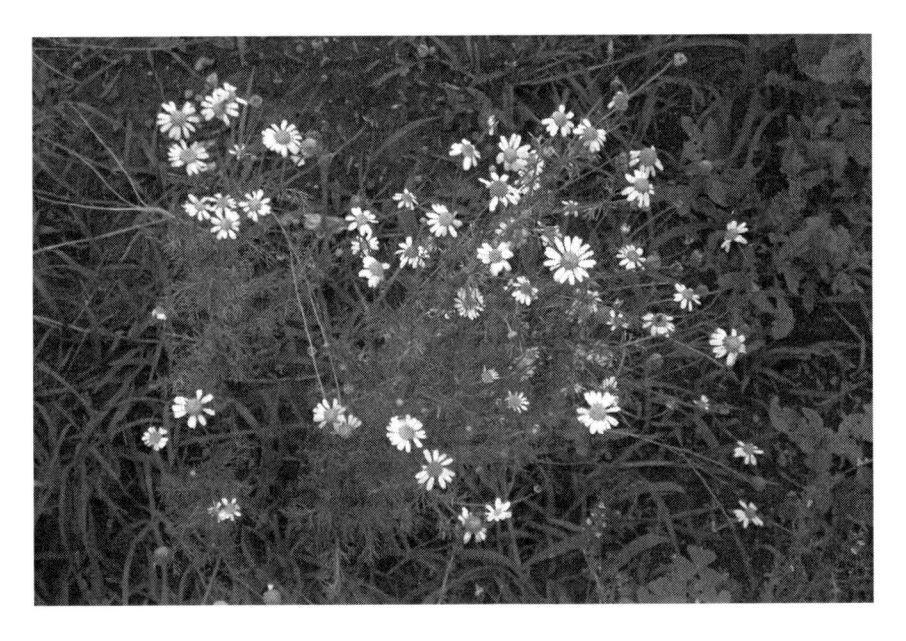

These are chamomile flowers growing in my backyard herb garden. I grow organic herbs and vegetables year-round. The herbs are used in salads, salad dressing, garnishes, and teas.

---

7   *The Green Pharmacy Herbal Handbook by James A. Duke, Ph.D.*

67   Rich Remedies

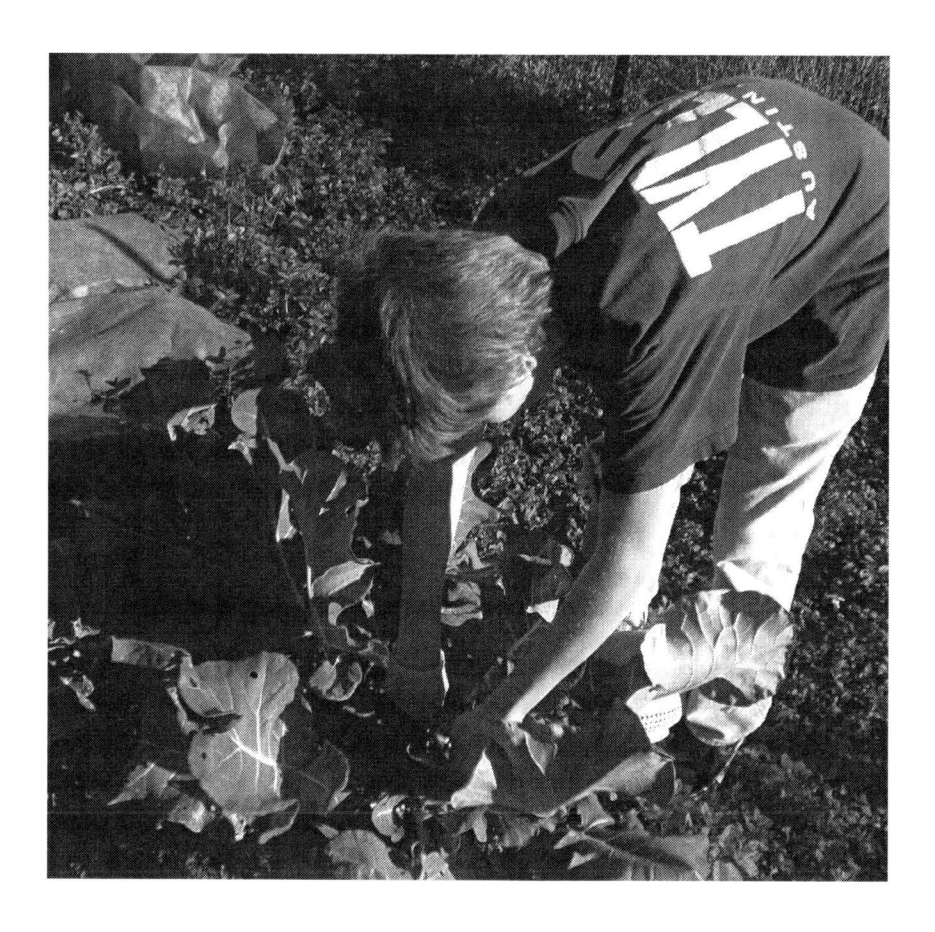

My son Christian harvesting fresh, organic herbs and broccoli from our backyard garden in the winter in Austin, Texas. We have a year-round growing season here in the Texas Hill Country so there are fresh garden vegetables on our table every month of the year. It's a nice feeling to grow your own food and eat it within minutes of being harvested. I fertilize with organic mulch, manure, and minerals including magnesium to insure that we get our daily allowance of this crucial mineral. In 2008 I introduced EM•1® Microbial Inoculants into the soil which will increase the life-giving properties of my soil with magnetic wave resonance.

Miraculous herb formula!

Ojibway Native American Remedy-Essiac

Rene Caisse, sometimes referred to as "Canada's Cancer Nurse," discovered a Native American remedy in 1922 that showed promise as a cure for cancer. The remedy is called Essiac (her last name spelled backwards), has been successfully used to treat hundreds of patients. This Ojibway Native American tribal concoction consists of burdock root, turkey rhubarb, sheep sorrel, and slippery elm. Caisse's clinic in Bracebridge, Ontario, Canada, was repeatedly attacked by the medical establishment and governmental bureaucrats. In spite of the pressure, she prevailed, saving many lives and improving the quality of life for cancer sufferers.

The story of her Essiac discovery goes something like this:

Caisse was nursing a woman in her 80s who had been admitted to a hospital in Ontario, Canada. She examined the woman and noticed that one of her breasts was deeply scarred and disfigured. Caisse asked the woman about her damaged breast. The woman told her that 20 plus years ago she had had breast cancer. She had gone to several doctors who had removed tumors from her breast, but they kept reappearing, ultimately being written off for dead by her physician.

She and her husband ran into a Native American Medicine Man who told them that he had an herbal tonic that would shrink and dissolve the tumors.

After having attempted to eliminate the breast tumors with conventional medicine, they reconnected with the Medicine Man in a last ditch, desperate attempt to heal her cancerous breast. She and her husband collected the prescribed herbs and mixed them in the recommended quantities. After taking the "medicine" for several months, the tumors in her breast shrank and disappeared.

Rich Remedies

Caisse used this remedy on many of the people that she encountered with cancer with miraculous results.

The herbs in the remedy exhibit healing qualities on their own, but it is thought that there is a synergistic effect when they are combined in the recommended quantities that create a total healing effect. Energetic *Resonance.*

Burdock root (*Arctium lappa*): Stimulates production of bile, helps liver function, acts as a blood purifier, has a reputation for tumor regression.

Turkey rhubarb (*Rheum pamatun*): Laxative, astringent, cleanses bowels, helps with liver toxicity.

Sheep sorrel (*Rumex acetosella*): High in vitamin C, diuretic helps in breaking down tumors.

Slippery elm (*Ulmus fulva*): Used to heal sore throats and wounds, and coat stomach and intestinal tract.

The Essiac Formula consists of 6 1/2 cups burdock root, 16 oz of powdered sheep sorrel, 1 oz. of Turkish rhubarb root powdered and 4 oz of slippery elm bark. These ingredients are mixed together and boiled in spring water to make a tea that is taken on an empty stomach each night before retiring.[8]

I have taken Essiac tea as a healing tonic several times just to try it out. (It tastes like dirt. Some may argue that dirt tastes better. They're pretty close in flavor so it's a hard call.) I felt fine, after I got past the taste, and it did make my digestive tract feel really good. This is something I intend to keep in my disease fighting arsenal. You can buy a six month supply that comes pre-made in plastic pouches for around $100.00. It keeps pretty well so I have it around for when I have the urge to take some, which isn't often. If I get the "BIG C",

---

[8] *For more information:http//www.essiacinfo.org*

this may be boiling on my stove every week! No guarantees, just an idea. Please consult your doctor for a full prescription.

These statements have not been evaluated by the Food and Drug Administration. This product is not intended to diagnose, treat, cure, or prevent disease.

Chapter 6
Internal Cleansing

For me, the most important discovery in the area of Nutrition

There are many different ways to cleanse your body: fasting, herbal tonics, electromagnetics, and colon hydrotherapy are four that I have used succesfully. Cleansing is important because our bodies accumulate environmental toxins and residues from a variety of sources which enter into and accumulate in the colon. If this stagnant accumulation is allowed to persist, it can become a major source of disease throughout our body since the colon is connected via nerves, to all areas. Nutrients and toxins are also absorbed into the blood stream through the colon. These facts were generally acknowledged long ago by me, but action was conveniently avoided for years until I was in my 40s and scared into action.

I'll go easy on you, in the beginning, and then work my way into the more challenging, yet most effective cleanses. So here's the easy stuff first.

Lemon water: Drinking the juice of a fresh lemon mixed with pure water is one of the simplest, yet effective cleanses you can employ on a daily basis. The yellow color of the lemon also improves your mood and has an alkalizing effect. Most people think lemons are acidic. They enter your body acidic but when digested turn alkaline because their ash is alkaline. Life is full of contradictions.

Ionized Water: A good water ionizer will purify and alkalize (raise the pH) level of your tap water. Drinking the recommended number of glasses of water (average 8 per day), is another good cleanser.

Internal Cleansing 72

This is covered in more detail in Chapter 18, Water as Medicine.

Q2 Energy Spa: This is an easy, simple, fast, and non-intrusive way to cleanse your body. Another form of bio-energetic therapy. I was introduced to this therapy in Albuquerque, NM. by Terry Kast, one of my healing coaches, who recommended that I "take the water" with this energetic therapy. There is a belief amongst Q2 users that its helps facilitate the removal of heavy metals from the body by generating negative ions that bind with the metal molecules in the blood stream.[9]

Heavy metals are one of the biggest silent killers. Mercury, lead, aluminum, cadmium, and arsenic are some of the common ones that are present everywhere in our environment. You cannot avoid consuming them therefore it is necessary to find a way to expel them from your body.

These metals accumulate in your body and literally short circuit your nervous system. Have you ever accidentally touched an electrical connection with metal and seen it spark? Have you ever short circuited the electricity in your house by overloading it? We are electrical beings. It's the same with our bodies. When you introduce metals into an electrical environment, the sparks fly. Destruction follows.

The presence of heavy metals in large quantities is linked to many illnesses. Mercury is present in many saltwater fish, vaccines, and amalgam tooth fillings. It is responsible for numerous neurological dysfunctions, including autism in children. Lead is in the atmosphere anywhere fossil fuels are being burned, in some glass containers, and glazed ceramics. Aluminum is in some kitchen cookware, deodorants, and beverage containers. It is linked to Alzheimer's disease by some medical practitioners.

Heavy metals can also be present in soil and water as a result of

---

9   *Q2 Energy Spa: www.Q2.com*

pollution and the use of chemical pesticides and fertilizers. Large-scale commercial farming has greatly increased their presence in our food supply. So the question to ask yourself is: How much heavy metal has accumulated in my body? Not "if" you have them. They're everywhere. There is no doubt, unless you choose to stick your head in a hole, as many of us do.

Removing heavy metals from your body is health-giving and boosts the immune system. Letting them accumulate can lead to numerous debilitating diseases over time. Chances are you'll have no idea of the source of your discomfort, since these invisible killers start short circuiting your nervous system, and neither will most of the doctors you see. They will most likely treat symptoms, but not recommend that you eliminate heavy metals from your body.

The Q2 Energy Spa is said to aid in heavy metal detoxification. The unit con¬sists of a control unit and a round ball with metal disks inside. You put the orb in a tub of water and then place your feet in the water. The electricity passing through the orb enters the water and resonates with the electric field in your body. It causes toxins and heavy metals to bind. They are then flushed out of your body through the liver and kidneys. You can feel the energy coursing through the water during the treatment. Following the treatments I felt relaxed and energized.

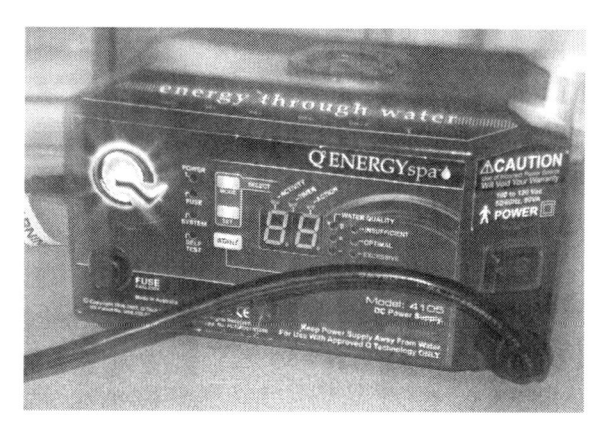

This is the Q Energy Spa Controller.

Internal Cleansing

The Q2 Energy Spa literature has loads of disclaimers in it about its healing benefits as do many bio-energetic devices not approved by the Food and Drug Administration (FDA). As with everything, get a healing coaches opinion and make your own judgment as to whether this cleansing tool will be beneficial to your health.

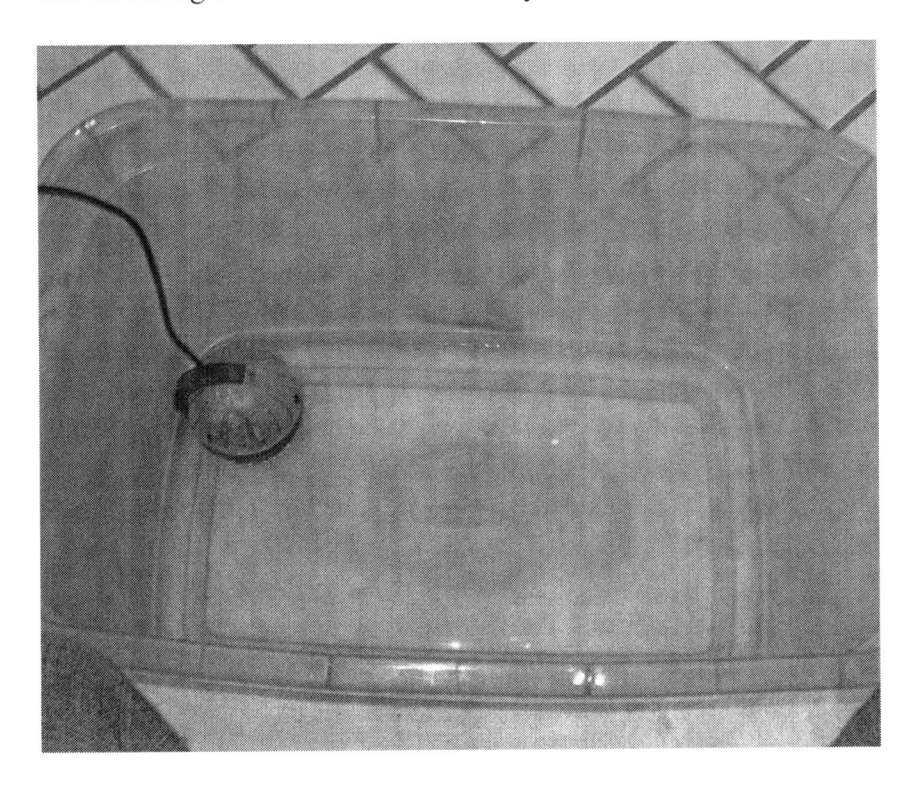

This is the Q2 energy Spa orb that contains magnets that send an energy charge through water in the tub into your feet, energizing the whole body.

Herbal cleanse

This is an herbal cleanse that I have used frequently to internally flush my system of toxic debris. It doesn't taste very good, but numerous people I know have ben-efitted from taking this.

Ingredients: Organic, unfiltered apple juice
Organic, unfiltered apple cider vinegar
Distilled water or purified water
Psyllium powder
Chickweed
Cinnamon
Powdered Ginger Root
Powdered black walnut hull (optional)

Instructions: 1. Take a containerr, fill with 8 oz apple juice, 8 oz of distilled water and 2–3 tablespoons of psyllium powder. Drink the solution quickly.

2. Fill the 32 oz jar with 16 oz distilled water, add 2 tablespoons of Apple Cider vinegar (or lemon juice). Add 1 teaspoon each of chickweed, cinnamon powder, ginger powder, and fennel powder. Shake well and drink solution.

Drink these solutions before lunch and late in the afternoon before dinner for five consecutive days. Try to refrain from drinking caffeine and alcohol. Avoid sugar and junk foods.

Friends and I have used this. We have all enjoyed weight loss, improved digestion, and a general feeling of well-being following its use. It's a little inconvenient, but it's worth the effort. There are many off the shelf herbal cleanses at health food stores that are easier to consume and just as effective as this one.

Consult your healing coach or physician before taking any cleanse. Do this under the supervision of a medical professional.

Colon Hydrotherapy

You will need to be shocked into getting a colonic. I was. This isn't for everyone, but it will deliver dramatic health-giving results, if you follow through with a program supervised by a trained, and certified colon hydro therapist. It will improve your mental and physical performance, as well as overall health.

I get a lot of flak from guys who hear that I do colon hydrotherapy. They look at me like I am some sort of odd ball. Let me set the record straight. If you are male or female and over 45 years of age, you are going to be directed by your family doctor to get a colonoscopy.

A colonoscopy is a long, thin tubular medical device with a camera, light, and with a cutter at the tip that is inserted into your anus and up into your colon. This is a diagnostic tool used to detect growths, such as polyps on the colon wall, or, in severe cases, cancerous tumors. If polyps are discovered they can be cut off with this device. If you are a "responsible" patient, you will have a colonoscopy done annually from the age of 45 until you die.

So those of you that think I'm weird for having a small plastic tube inserted into me …

I'm approaching the same problem you are, but as preventative medicine, and from a different angle and using a different process. Same church … different pew. The buttocks are always a sensitive subject. Must be that it is the root chakra? (According to Eastern philosophy, the basis of all of your earthly emotional issues is tied to the "root chakra".)

Colon hydrotherapy came to my attention after a friend got severe food poisoning in a New York City sushi restaurant in 2004. He got severe abdominal cramps, fever, and passed out. He was taken to the emergency ward of a nearby hospital and admitted. The doctors performed tests and administered IV fluids. He was fed a massive quantity of the antibiotic, Cipro (I am a big fan of Cipro™, when used properly) and sent on his way.

When he got back home to Austin, Tex., he was run through a battery of tests during which they happened to find a lump on one of his lungs. They could not tell if it was cancer or a benign growth, so they told him that they would need to monitor it for the next year. Cancer was a possibility.

Naturally, as soon as the term "Cancer" is brought into a conversation, we all freak out. You may as well say "death" because that is the connotation cancer has with most of us. (My perspective on cancer has changed since this scare, but at the time I freaked. I'm less worried about it now since I think there are a number of non-painful ways that it can be overcome.)

I gave my buddy some advice (go alkaline, cancer thrives in an acidic environment) and directed him to a few websites to check out natural cures and getting alkaline. Also suggested that he visit a holistic healing professional. On his own he found a few natural healing websites that graphically showed how acidosis comes about and described what goes on in your digestive system when acidic, undigested foods accumulate. He sent me multiple web links to holistic healing sites.

One web site that he sent me had vivid photos and descriptions of putrefied feces in intestines that absolutely disgusted me. I could not disassociate my insides from the photos of these slimy monsters that were extracted from sick people's colons. (See Dr. Bernard Jensen's book *Guide to Better Bowel Care* for photos.) This stuff is absolutely revolting. As hard as I tried, I could not erase the images from my mind, so I decided to expunge whatever vile slop I had collected over 40 plus years from my body. It became a crusade.

Like me, you have accumulated this slime from years as the result of eating the American diet and being subjected to environmental toxins.

This toxic slurry is leaching poison, heavy metals, chemicals, acids, filth, carcinogens, and other toxins into your bloodstream through the lining of your colon, the same way food nutrients are assimilated. When it gets dense enough and caked onto the walls of your colon, it blocks the absorption of healthy nutrients by the body, often causing malnutrition and auto-intoxication.

Hey I know this isn't fun, but it's true. Don't shoot the messenger. I'm just telling you what's going on in the deepest, darkest confines of your body. It ain't pretty!

As you can imagine, this darkness creates an acidic, anaerobic, oxygen-starved environment where deadly parasites and cancerous cells thrive. They love it here! It's hell on earth and they can't get enough of this filth. The payback for generously providing this refuge: irritable bowel syndrome, candida, vaginitis, colon cancer, and all other sicknesses.

To prepare myself for this cleansing journey, I went out and bought a copy of Dr. Jensen's classic book on the subject. Dr. Jensen was a Chiropractor who, based on his training, focused on the spine, the central highway of the nervous system, as the center of all cures and a central point for healing. However, Dr. Jenson got sick and could not cure his problem with his chiropractic training. As a result, he discovered and addressed his issue by removing the blockage in his colon. This changed the way he approached healing. Additionally, Dr. Jensen was one of America's foremost pioneering experts in the field of nutrition, mentoring many of today's best practitioners in the field of Naturopathy. One of his best known accomplishments was in the field of iridology, the study of the eye to determine tissue weakness and imbalances in the body. He operated Hidden Valley Ranch in Escondido, Cal., as a wellness center from 1955 until his death in 2001.

I discovered three things in Dr. Jensen's book that were profound to me: (1) cell death is due to an autointoxication process that starts in the bowel, (2) the neural arc reflex defines the connection of the bowel wall to the entire nervous system, and (3) the fact that most, if not all, disease starts in the bowel.[10] You can heal just about any illness, if you take care of your digestive system, in particular, your colon.

The remedy for most health issues starts with bowel care and *Dr. Jensen's Seven Day Cleanse*, which includes colon hydrotherapy. Unless you are really serious about getting healthy, you probably do not need to proceed further. Thus stuff is not hard, "butt"

---

10 Jensen, Bernard. *Dr. Jensen's Guide to Better Bowel Care.* New York: Avery, Penguin Putman, 1999. Page 86.

uncomfortable for most people.

Before delving into colon hydrotherapy lets briefly discuss the three discoveries that I found profound in Dr. Jensen's work.

Dr. Jensen tells of Alex Carrel, MD, a Nobel Prize winning physician, who in 1912, proved that heart cells from a chicken embryo could be kept alive almost indefinitely, by simply keeping the solution they were in clean and by providing the proper nutrients.[11] The cells were kept alive in his laboratory for 29 years and died only because one day a nurse forgot to clean the solution. I'm told that the average lifespan of a chicken is less than six years due to Colonel Sanders, raccoons, opossums, foxes, disease, and neighborhood dogs. In the absence of these predators, a chicken lives less than 10 years. These cells survived approximately 19 years past a normal chicken's life, or three times the lifespan of your average lucky chicken. The cells died of autointoxication, the same process that causes us to get sick and die. Like the chicken cells, our cells die when they are polluted by the waste products in our bodies. This occurs primarily from toxins leaching into our bloodstream through the walls of the colon. So, by extension, if you keep the toxins minimized in your colon, you will minimize the toxins and carcinogens in your blood stream. Make sense?

The second revelation was that of neural arc reflex, a term Dr. Jensen coined to describe the direct connection that exists between your colon and the nerves that connect it to your entire body. (This is akin to the meridian connections used in traditional Chinese medicine.) The interesting part of this is that Dr. Jensen discovered that there is a reflexive or direct connection between the bowel and our other organs. If you cleanse or relieve the area of the bowel that corresponds to the liver, the liver gets better; the same is true with your arms, legs, heart, kidneys, and other areas of your body.

A common example of how this works is illustrated by people who are admitted to the emergency ward of the hospital with severe

---

11 Jensen, Bernard. *Dr. Jensen's Guide to Better Bowel Care.* New York: Avery, Penguin Putman, 1999. Page 43.

chest pains and have a simulated heart attack. This happens all the time. The source of the "heart attack" is the bowel, not the heart. Its neurological impulse, caused by "putrefactive debris" in the colon, transmits an aberrant nerve signal to the heart. Thus, indigestion is a blockage or lack of flow; a blockage of ki. These heart attack-like episodes are quite common and can be prevented by proper bowel care. This phenomenon is known as referred pain.[12] I know a lot of people who suffer from **referred pain**. They have no idea what causes it and pound away at their symptoms with their doctor's help and prescription drugs, instead of addressing the source of their problem which is their bowel.

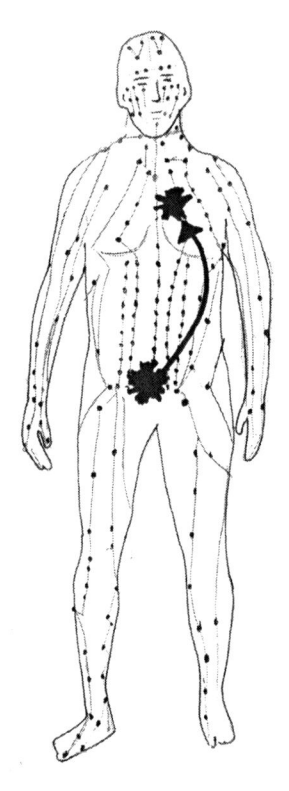

This is a simple illustration of the illusive concept of referred pain.

---

12 Jensen, Bernard. *Dr. Jensen's Guide to Better Bowel Care.* New York: Avery, Penguin Putman, 1999. Page 88.

You think you're having a heart attack, when in reality you have an intestinal block.

I know many people who have gone to the hospital emergency ward with chest pains who thought they were in cardiac arrest. In many cases they were suffering from intestinal blockage, or referred pain. So keep your digestive tract unobstructed, clear and healthy and you may be able to avoid this inconvenience.

If you're reading this… now you know. Joint pain, muscle aches, headaches, abdominal pain, you name it, the origin is probably in your colon, believe it or not. Dare to give yourself an enema like my granny gave me when I was 4 years old. The pain goes away. Like the good old days before we had over-the-counter BS for everything. Big Pharma has banished this healing modality from our consciousness and has made it a source of collective embarrassment.

The third revelation was that almost every illness has its origin in the bowel. Take care of the bowel first. You would be amazed at the number of things that you'll cure cleansing the bowel. As unpopular a subject as this is, it is an "inconvenient truth."[13] Sorry Al, this pithy line relates as well here to the bowel as it does to your reference to global warming…I couldn't resist.…I had to use it.

So, after gaining a full appreciation for the role of the colon in health, I decided to take the plunge and do the Dr. Jensen Seven Day Cleanse which includes colon hydrotherapy. The cleanse consists of taking drinks of distilled water, apple juice, psyllium, apple cider vinegar, vegetable broth, and a whole slew of vitamins and minerals, while avoiding solid foods, for a week.

Colon Hydrotherapy, or Colonics for short, is a process where approximately 12 gallons of body temperature (approximately 100 degrees) water is gradually pumped through a tube into your rectum and colon, under light pressure, for about 35 to 40 minutes. This process causes fecal matter stuck to the walls of the colon to fall off and flow into a holding tank (sewer) below the machine. (It takes

---

13 Jensen, Bernard. *Dr. Jensen's Guide to Better Bowel Care.* New York: Avery, Penguin Putman, 1999. Page 86.

multiple sessions to clean years of residual, hardened feces from the intestinal wall.) To be most effective, colonics is usually done in conjunction with an herbal, or tonic, cleanse to help loosen things up.

Sounds like fun campers, doesn't it? Who wants to volunteer to sit on the throne first?

My Experience

This is in my top three measures for wellness. It took me 48 years to do this and I wish I had done this sooner, but everything has its time.

You will need to be shocked into getting a colonic. I was. Most people will never do something like this and I do understand completely your personal phobias. This is not for everybody, unless you are really serious about cleansing your body and being disease free. If you have a death wish, by all means, don't do this as it will likely extend your life.

Earlier in the book I said that many illnesses originate in the mind due to stress and toxic thoughts. I will extend this to say that, if the toxic thoughts don't kill you, the toxic chemicals that accumulate in your colon, your own personal, private, in-body septic system, will. Yes, your "Uncle Jessie"," Aunt Bessy, and my great-grandfather lived to 93 without this fancy crap. But they did not live in the same world that we live in today. Their food was fresher and the environment was less toxic. When my grand pappy grew up there was no fast food. Plastics, pesticides, agricultural chemicals, population growth, nuclear testing, increased electromagnetic frequencies, artificial foods, and many other factors contribute to the toxicity in our lives-were not around. Our times are different.

So how did I get into this?

My friend's cancer scare, and some small lingering traces of asthma after I completed the Blood Type Diet, convinced me that the time had come in my life for a complete oil change. I was beginning to write this book and thought it would make a great chapter. Dr. Jensen's revelations on the colon being the center of my universe also convinced me this was worth doing.

I try to explain colon hydrotherapy this way: "The reason that the bowel needs to be cleansed is the same reason you have the "honey wagon" show up to your house to empty the septic system. You don't want all that "grease" backing up in your toilets and spilling all over your yard and house. Do you? So you don't want this happening in your body either. In effect, when your colon gets clogged, toxins leach through the colon wall and cause intestinal toxemia and autointoxication. It's self poisoning.

The same thing that happens to your house happens in your body if your colon is not flushed. Fecal matter, mucus, undigested pills, chemicals, sugars, parasites, yeasts, molds, micro toxins, and other harmful agents accumulate in the colon, rot, then leach into your bloodstream. The poisons in your colon are carried to all parts of your body where they find a resting place in your organs, muscles, lymph, and then skin. Your cells end up bathing in poison, which weakening them making them susceptible to disease. This is auto intoxication or simply self-poisoning. You also experience referred pain. As the poisons build up in your colon, they weaken the immune system, cells, and organs, brain...the entire body. This state of "healthy sickness" is the breeding ground and gateway for anger, cancer, heart disease, multiple sclerosis, influenza, parasites, and all the other things that make you sick.

Another complication is the impaction of fecal matter, which also prevents food nutrients from leaching into your bloodstream because the pathway is blocked. (Isn't this a delightful subject? Don't you just love this book?)

The American fast food diet is one of the main culprits of bowel disease. Pasty unrefined white flour, French fries, refined sugars, tainted meat, and processed foods all contribute to malfunctions of the colon. Add to this pharmaceuticals, over-the-counter medicines, household chemicals and cleansers, environmental pollution, and television (I had to throw this in here) and it's no wonder health costs in America are out of control.

A healthy diet of fresh, organic vegetables, produce, and clean water will substantially reduce the conditions I describe here. People who have high fiber, vegetable-based diets rarely have diabetes, appendicitis, diverticulitis, polyps, or cancer of the colon.

Even if you have a healthy diet, you will ingest environmental toxins that will need to be flushed.

Okay! Quit right here! Order an extra large pepperoni pizza with sausage and anchovies. Indulge while you can. And order a six pack of Old Milwaukee beer while you're at it. Knock yourself out!

I guarantee that most of you have this toxic soup in your body. It is leaching poison, heavy metals, chemicals, acids, carcinogens, and other toxins into your bloodstream, through the lining of your colon, the same way food nutrients are assimilated. When it gets dense enough and caked on the walls of your colon, it blocks the absorption of healthy nutrients, causing malnutrition.

Here is a short list of common environmental toxins that you may be storing and absorbing: dioxin, mercury, lead, cadmium, arsenic, aluminum, PCBs, carbon monoxide, pharmaceuticals, food-based chemicals, and any chemicals that you come in daily contact with.

Like me, many of you will point out that your great-grandfather was a genetic miracle and a statistical anomaly who lived to be 93 years old even though he smoked two packs of unfiltered cigarettes a day, drank a six pack of crummy beer daily, and ate nothing but meat, preferably pork since he was a good German-American. Everybody has a person that they use to reinforce their own behavior and give themselves a sense of immortality. It's human nature. I do it.

Very few people can abuse themselves like this and get away with it for 93 years, but we all have our examples of the relative who beat all the odds and did not die screaming in some old folks' home with a tube in their throat and someone's finger in a dark space. I hope that we are part of this elite group of statistical anomalies who beat the nursing home torture. Most of us who live that long will experience these indignities, unless we do something about it. I'm trying to help you…see?

The Process

The colon hydrotherapy machine is a reclining fiberglass sofa-like chair with a whole, drain, and tube located where you buttocks rests. You sit or lie back and insert a plastic tube into your butt about 3 inches. (Not the 12 inches the colonoscopy requires.) Water at body temperature (approximately 100 degrees) is slowly pumped through the tube into your bowel cavity. The bowel fills up, contracts, and pushes fecal matter out into the drain below.

The model I used actually had a clear, plastic tube for viewing the grease as it is flowing into the sewer system below. You can watch a life time's worth of impacted, putrefied, undigested food get flushed out of your body and in many cases see some of your sicknesses washed away after multiple sessions. It really sounds disgusting, doesn't it? I agree, but what's worse, flushing it out or carrying that disease-breeding muck around with you inside your body for the rest of your life? Most people will refuse to acknowledge that they have a rotting sewer in their belly. Not me, I admit it and get on with cleansing it on a regular basis. It's my "oil change."

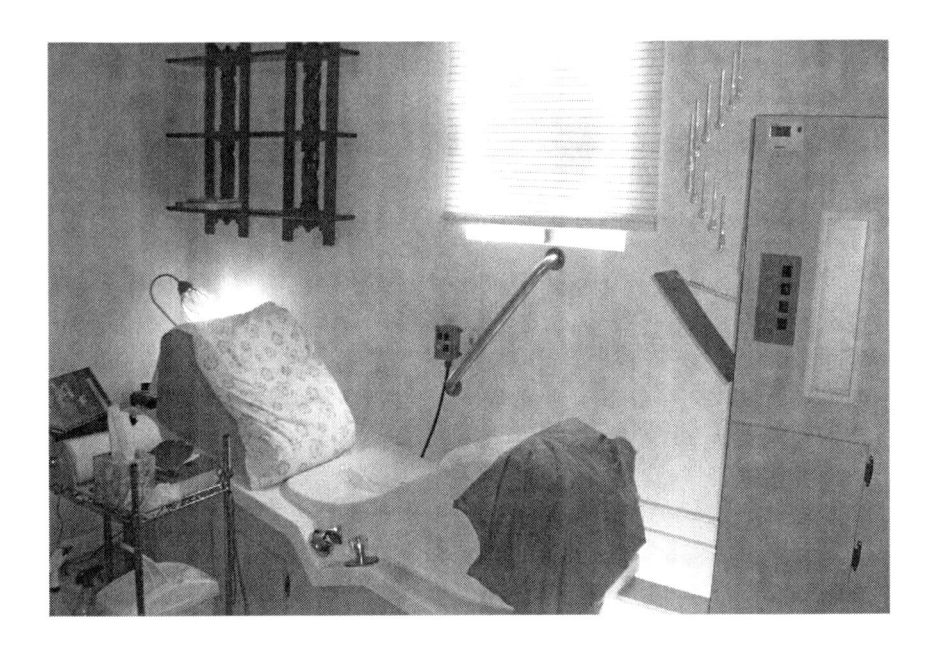

This is the colon hydrotherapy equipment that I used under the direction of a certified colon hydro therapist. You can see the "thrown" that you recline on to the left and the vertical water tank on the right. Once you get your mind past this whole process, the end result of the cleanse is worth it.

Results

I have cured eczema, asthma, and allergies and lost crappy weight, and I believe that it helped to reduce my cholesterol. My eyesight has improved and my sense of taste and smell skyrocketed. I guess that I have reduced my chronological age by about ten years by slowing down the cell death caused by autointoxication. (This last point is my unscientific opinion.)

Other conditions that may benefit from colon hydrotherapy are: MS, Candida, fibromyalgia, arthritis, and any toxic-shock based illness where poisons have accumulated in the colon causing severe sickness.

I can confirm Dr. Jensen's premise that everything starts with the colon.

If you are an adventurous spirit and want to experience some significant improvements in your health, consult a naturopath about colon hydrotherapy and a Seven Day Cleanse. For some people this is life changing. In addition to cleaning out your body, metaphorically it cleanses you of old, worn out beliefs, bad memories and bad habits. For me there was an unprecedented sense of clarity.

SECTION 2
ENERGY MEDICINE—MOVING ENERGY

Chapter 7
Acupuncture

Acupuncture is an ancient Chinese healing method that is believed to have been founded over 3,000 years ago. It and other meridian-focused healing arts are based on the theory that the body has an energy force running through it. This energy force is known as Ki includes all life activities, i.e., spiritual, emotional, mental, and physical, while working in combination with the universal forces of yin and yang (the harmony of opposites). According to traditional Chinese medicine, when there are blockages of the pathways, yin and yang are thrown out of balance causing sickness and disease.

Chi, Ki, Qi, and prana come from air, water, and food. Chi is "bionic" or "bioelectric energy. This combines the idea of living organisms (bio) with that of electric and negatively charged ions (ionic). French scientist. J. Belot, PhD said, "When we consider organic life in the light of biophysics, we find that electrical phenomena are at the root of all cellular life and we conclude that the end of everything is an electrical charge."[1]

Ki travels along meridians (energy channels). There are fourteen pairs running through the body and twelve of those connect with vital organs. The meridians run up and down the surface of the body acting as pathways for energy and have specific acupuncture points. (Other terms for these are target or potent points.)

The acupuncturists insert needles into these points at angles between 15 degrees and 90 degrees

The most common ailments that acupuncture is said to treat are: asthma, headaches, allergies, arthritic conditions, alcohol abuse,

---

[1] Dr. J. Belot PhD. copied with permission from www.waterworks4u.com. Benefits of Ionized water.

smoking, and drug addiction. There are others, but these are the ones that I have heard most frequently mentioned. In the section on AcuScen, "Acupuncture on Steroids" you will see that acupuncture has been taken to a whole new level with sophisticated technology that heals many diseases.

My Experience

I have used acupuncture on multiple occasions. The first time I used it was when a healing catalyst was needed to speed my recovery from an acute ear and throat infection that had lasted four weeks and had me on two separate regimens of antibiotics. I turned to acupuncture because I could not shake the sickness and was getting worried that it was slowly killing me. (The illness had an intelligence that I could sense.) It was attacking me from multiple angles: sleep deprivation, insomnia, heavy uncontrollable coughing that brought on severe headaches, ringing in my ears, and swollen glands. The discomfort was continuous. I had the worst thick phlegm (mucus), weakness, and was losing my hearing as the congestion migrated to the inner ear.

Cipro™, a powerful antibiotic, was prescribed and clearly attacked the infection effectively, helping me conquer it. (Never let it be said that I do not appreciate prescription drugs. They have their place in healing. I just don't appreciate the unnecessary prescriptions and manipulation of our system by big pharma.) During the treatment of this sickness, I believe the acupuncture aided in the improvement of my circulation and helped remove the blocked pathways in my body.

The acupuncture process was painless and relaxing. After the acupuncturist discussed the nature of the problem, needles were inserted at points along the meridians that would impact the area that needed healing. When the needles were inserted I noticed a buzzing, vibrating sensation at the top of some of the needles. Detectable energy was flowing through my body. This is not a sensation that I can easily describe, but it was invigorating. It was a full body buzz that felt very energizing in a good way. I had five treatments, the minimum recommended by my acupuncturist to have a therapeutic effect. Some Chinese herbs were also prescribed, and acidophilus for post-antibiotic treatment of my intestinal flora.

I cannot determine with certainty exactly what the acupuncture accomplished. My energy level picked up during this time, which I believe increased my body's ability to fight bacterial infection in concert with the antibiotics. Sleep improved the night after each treatment. My intuition tells me it worked, I just can't pinpoint how.

My second major acupuncture experience came early in the winter of 2003. Cedar allergy season erupted in Austin, sending my body full tilt into allergic reaction culminating in an upper respiratory infection and asthma. My realtor told me that she had cured her cedar allergies 100%, after suffering for years, by getting acupuncture treatments. On this advice I researched acupuncturists in Austin and selected one whom I felt had the most experience and best credentials. In addition to ten acupuncture treatments, Chinese herbs were prescribed to assist in the cedar allergy treatment.

During the course of this therapy, I experienced a "healing crisis" that included severe headaches, sinus pain, upset stomach, and sleeplessness. (Sometimes your affliction needs to get worse before it gets better.) However, after the crisis, my allergy symptoms improved- and then got worse again. I went back to my doctor who prescribed antibiotics, steroids, and an inhaler. As with my first experience, the acupuncture delivered energy improving benefits, but no immediate or obvious relief from allergies and the asthma.

My acupuncturist told me that approximately 10% of patients get little or no benefit from acupuncture. I may be a ten percenter, although the healing may have been delayed in my case. The vast majority of people with whom I speak say acupuncture has had profound positive results on allergies and other ailments.

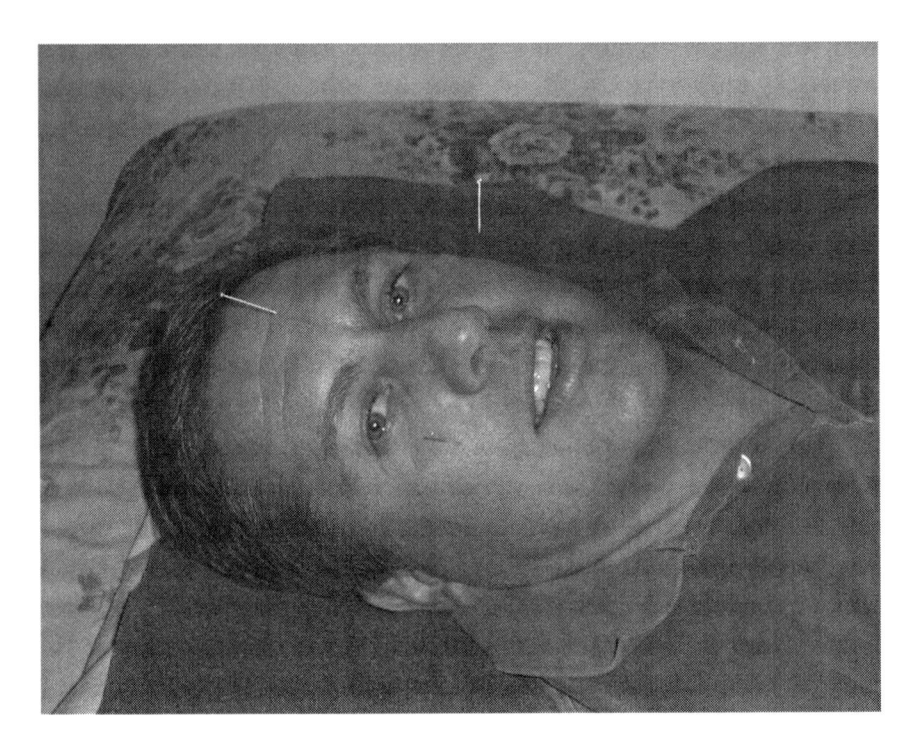

The author with Acupuncture needles inserted in the face (and other areas not seen in this photo) to treat allergies and asthma. The Acupuncture did facilitate energy clearing/healing, but the final resolution to my problems came through nutritional supplements and a diet that restricted certain allergy-causing foods as well as internal cleansing. My healing coaches for allergy resolution included an Acupuncturist, a certified nutritionist, colon hydro therapist, then threw in my own personal research into all of these areas so that I completely understood what was being done to me.

Chapter 8
Acupuncture on Steroids

AcuScen or Self Controlled Energo-Neuro-Adaptive Regulation (SCENAR) "Fast, Space Age Chinese Medicine"

Imagine yourself hurtling through outer space at three times the speed of sound looking down at the blue and white sphere of earth, flying 250 miles above the surface. You are in a sealed tube for at least seven days orbiting the earth, when you get sick. Another seven days stand between you and a doctor on Earth. There is a modest selection of medicine from which to choose. What do you do so far from home, in space? This is the problem that the Soviet space program and the Cosmonaut Training Center wished to tackle in the 1980s. They were looking for a drugless remedy for healing in outer space.

Russian scientist, Alexander Karasev, had been working on an electronic immune system stimulator called SCENAR (Self Controlled Energo-Neuro-Adaptive Regulation) at the Cosmonaut Training Center. Karasev took the SCENAR technology and refined it over the years, producing a tool that has delivered amazing healing results. (The Soviets used a variation of Karasev's invention in space with modest success.)

My introduction to this technology was through SCENAR's successor technology called AcuScen. I like to think of AcuScen (SCENAR) as accelerated intelligent electrical acupuncture. Like acupuncture it leverages traditional Chinese energy medicine using the meridians and potent points to send stimulation to the brain and nervous system.

In simple terms, it works like this:

The AcuScen is a battery powered hand-held device that is placed on the skin in the area of pain, or potent point that is associated with a distressed organ (example of "referred pain"). It sends a constantly varying electrical signal to the brain triggering instructions to the nervous system which then produces neuropeptides, the body's healing chemicals. The AcuScen enables the brain to break through energy blockages promoting healing. Similar to acupuncture, the patient can get immediate relief, or it can take a series of treatments to resolve the issue, depending on the individual's receptivity and the advancement of the illness.

AcuScen has a very sophisticated software program that senses and measures the electrical activity of the body and then automatically adjusts the frequency to correct imbalances. This is biofeedback or bio-energy at work. The electrical impulse AcuScen sends out copies the body's own energy signals instructing the brain and body to generate the specific peptides needed for healing. It has a real-time biofeedback loop that varies the electrical impulses and learns from each succeeding series of stimulus. The treatment seeks to break energy blocks, balancing the yin and yang in the body.

My Experience

I am always in search of the "magic healing bullet," even though I know a single "bullet" does not exist. AcuScen is most certainly one of the top remedies I will keep in my healing tool box.

This concept of using electric pulses to heal is not new to me. I sustained damage to my left knee in a skiing accident in Colorado about ten years ago. It was the last ski run of the day on a Sunday. I had been skiing hard for three days and was exhausted. My friend Bill, who lives in Colorado and used to ski at least thirty times per season, decided to take me through a glade of aspen trees and large boulders next to a triple diamond, expert ski run called Palvacini; a very steep, very narrow, and very treacherous run. (Part of the trail also winds under the ski lift so you have the ski lift utility poles to contend with in addition to the other hazards.) On my fearful descent through the narrow glade of trees, I face planted into a snow bank trying to avoid a collision with a tree stump. I twisted and banged my knee causing inflammation and bruising. The knee swelled up making it difficult to put weight on it.

A few days after the fall, a doctor examined my knee and suggested that an orthopedic surgeon have a look. Around this time I ran into a friend who had just used electrical therapy to heal a sports injury he had recently sustained. He referred me to a Naturopath who used an electric pulse machine to assist in mending moderate trauma and muscle injuries. Against the advice of my wife and close friends, I decided to skip the orthopedic specialist and experiment with the electric therapy. (Probably a dumb idea, but I was willing to experiment with alternative therapy and use the orthopedic doctor as my backup, plan should the electrical stimulation fail to do the job.)

The doctors I chose were an Indian couple who had set up shop in a big old, early 1900s stone house in the Overbrook section of West Philadelphia. I was greeted at the door by the husband (who looked malnourished, as do many vegetarians) and escorted to the dark semi-finished basement. The minute I walked into the basement I knew this was going to be a weird experience. In addition to me, there were four or five elderly people, who looked half dead, hooked up to intravenous drips. It was explained to me that they were heart patients who had so much plaque built up in their arteries that they were getting emergency Chelation Therapy as no heart surgeon would operate due to their weakened states. (This whole scene weirded me out. It was like a haunted house!)

ChelationTherapy is an intravenous drip of healing nutrients sent directly into the patient's blood stream for maximum effectiveness. I've never tried it, but there are a lot of people out there who have extended their lives by cleaning out their clogged arteries using this therapy.

The husband side of this doctor duo sat me down in a chair and hooked me up to a box with knobs and dials on it that looked like something you would use to tune up a car. Electrodes with suction cups were positioned around my swollen knee cap. The device is called an Eletro Acuscope. I felt a mild burning sensation on my skin at each contact point beneath the electrodes as the machine was activated. The electric juice was turned on and the electric current adjusted to just below the point of causing me discomfort.

The treatments, which were administered once a day for two weeks, completely healed my damaged knee. The pain and swelling went away in the first week of treatment and I got back full use of my left leg within ten days. As a result of this experience, healing a sports injury with electricity in a non-conventional way, AcuScen makes total sense to me.

I came across AcuScen technology quite by accident (as with many of the treatments in this book) and believe that the potential benefits are much greater, than what is expressing here.

A friend of mine in Austin had an interest in energy healing, and was looking to expand a naturopathic healing practice with the addition of AcuScen. As part of this effort, she hosted a three day training seminar with Mikhail Teppone, MD, a world-renowned authority in Extremely High Frequency (EHF) therapy, Chinese medicine, and acupuncture. Dr. Teppone and his partners in Ontario, Canada have advanced the original SCENAR technology and incorporated its advanced functions into the AcuScen device. (AcuScen is state-of-the art SCENAR technology.) He treads cautiously when discussing the full potential of AcuScen so as not to upset the AMA and FDA, who are always looking to shut down alternative therapies in the name of consumer protection.

Dr. Teppone started his career in allopathic medicine, but was drawn to the power and efficacy of natural Chinese healing methods. Having been on both sides he can speak with authority on the advantages of this natural healing method. Dr. Teppone is my model of what a physician should be. He has the knowledge and training of a conventional medical doctor, combined with expertise in Chinese medicine, so he can offer the best of both worlds. He does not dismiss any healing technique, sharing my opinion that, the technique that works best for the individual is the right technique, irrespective of what it is. Most medical doctors look to surgery and pharmaceuticals for the cure. I think it's best to start with the least intrusive, natural remedy and then work your way into the heavy stuff.

What I found in speaking with him was that conventional medicine and drugs are rarely needed if a patient uses AcuScen and Chinese medicine. Invasive surgeries, toxic chemical therapies, and expensive pharmaceutical prescriptions can very often be avoided under the care of a trained AcuScen therapist who is also trained in Chinese medicine.

My personal exposure to AcuScen has been limited to the self administered treatments received at the Austin seminar and the research that I have done on the subject. At the time of the seminar I had a heavily bruised, swollen, injured thumb that was treated with the AcuScen device. My thumb responded quite well to the short duration electric stimulation and was completely healed within a week.

The AcuScen has been used successfully in sports medicine to accelerate the healing of torn muscles and tendons and multiple stress-related injuries. A well-known Tour de France Champion is rumored to have been treated extensively with AcuScen to heal faster and to provide an "unfair," but perfectly legal, edge over the competition. (This occurs due to the energetic intelligence intrinsic in the AcuScen device in the hands of a trained practitioner. It pinpoints areas of trauma and sends frequencies that aid in repairing damaged tissue).

I am really pumped about AcuScen but due to my limited personal exposure I have asked Dr. Teppone to share some of his first-hand success with a few representative case studies.

Here are a few of Dr. Teppone's "real-world" stories of AcuScen healing:

Patient 1 had very **intensive low back pain**, which appeared after lifting a heavy suitcase. Extremely High Frequency (EHF) therapy or "Needle free acupuncture" was applied with the Artsakh device just in the very beginning. During treatment intensity of the pain initially increased, then decreased and disappeared completely.[1]

Patient 2 had a **frozen shoulder**. This female patient had a pain in her right shoulder. This pained aggravated gradually during five years. All conventional and alternative treatments she took were not effective. I applied AcuScen device on the painful site on the shoulder and along her right arm. Additionally needling of the 1st point of Large Intestine meridian on the opposite site was applied. After this one session pain almost has gone and the patient began to move her right hand as well her left hand for the first time in years".

Patient 3, a female patient, 67, had a severe **phantom pain** after amputation of her leg. We provided Acupressure of the point Sp-4 (Gong Sun) connected to Chong May Extra channel on the healthy side. After a short time, her pain increased dramatically, the phantom pain suddenly vanished and has not appeared again. Author's note: She experienced a "healing crisis" whereby the condition gets worse before it gets better. The body breaks the blocked Ki, creates pain and then relief.

Patient 4, a male patient, 36, had a terminal stage **Hodgkin's disease**. During twelve years of disease he had received more than fifteen courses of chemotherapy and X-ray therapy as well. He went from bad to worse. During the first month of EHF-therapy his condition

---

1 Summary provided by Dr. Mikhail Teppone, MD, 2007

became stable. After next two months all symptoms of the disease had disappeared. Later he received several courses of needle-free acupuncture to support his health. He lived an additional four years in spite of a diagnosis that had determined he had no more time to live.

Patient 5, a male patient, 78, had a relapse of skin **Melanoma cancer** with metastasis into the brain. He received surgical operation and about 10 courses of chemotherapy and X-ray therapy. Nevertheless, the prognosis for his disease still was very bad and they suggested a dismal end in a month or two. In 2001, after assessment with ANTEL software he began to receive EHF-therapy and Moxibustion. Now [2007] his condition is stable and he is continuing to apply Moxibustion himself.[2]

Patient 6, a male patient, 45, with decomposition of **gastro-duodenal** stenosis had his schedule for surgical operation in a month. He received four sessions of EHF-therapy. In a month all symptoms of stenosis had gone and endoscopic examination revealed significant improvement of gastro-duodenal permeability. A surgeon did not recommend doing operation at that time. He was apparently healed.

Additional Successes

Gastric polyps: Extremely High Frequency (EHF) Puncture can be used successfully in treating patients with gastric polyps. After 1–4 months of treatment, besides clinical improvement, it is possible to achieve disappearance or diminution of gastric polyps ..." [M. Teppone. Therapeutic Effect of EHF-Puncture on Gastric Polyps. Amer. J. Acupuncture, 1991, 19 (1): 11–16.].

Peptic ulcers: Extremely high frequency (EHF) radiation was performed in 95 outpatients with duodenal ulcer. Individual choice of the exposure site can improve the treatment results. The syndrome-oriented approach of the Chinese conventional medicine warrants an effective choice of the acupuncture loci and the prognosis of the outcome. A clinical syndrome was identified in which healing of the ulcer was achieved on week two of the treatment in 92.3 +/- 7.7% of the patients. [M. Teppone, et al. Ultrahigh frequency therapy of duodenal ulcer—Klin Med (Moscow), 1991 Oct; 69 (10): 74–78: PMID: 1766225].

More Results from the SCENAR technology and AcuScen

In Russia, some 600 practitioners currently use the SCENAR, or AcuScen technology, as their principal treatment instrument, with over 50,000 reported cases of individual use. Their athletes have been known not only to compete after serious injuries, but even to break world-records post-SCENAR therapy. Russian accident and emergency wards, utilize the technology to aid recovery from cardiac arrest, massive trauma and coma. Finally, trials in Russia have also realized SCENAR's usage for pain management, with both cancer and fracture patients, finding more relief with the release of natural opioids after SCENAR treatment than from those externally administered.

A vast wealth of information on it is available from research papers, clinical reports and training manuals. It can be used on most types of disease or injury: circulatory, sensory, respiratory, neurological, genito-urinary, musculoskeletal, gastro-intestinal, endocrine, immune and psychological disorders and is credited with vastly reducing recovery times.

AcuScen Operation

The AcuScen is run over the spine and abdomen or infected area. The software records the resistive response to its signals and returns

---

2 All passages, courtesy of Dr. Mikhail Teppone, MD, AcuScen Inventor, Researcher, a and Medical Doctor.2007.

a fresh signal, causing a gentle tingling or stroking sensation. The practitioner is looking for anomalies on the skin surface, which may be highlighted by redness, numbness, or stickiness, or a change in the numerical display or sound. Although these areas may not seem to directly relate to the obvious symptoms, by treating these 'asymmetries' (as the Russians call them) with the AcuScen, the healing process will commence. A chronic problem may require up to six weeks of treatment, with long-lasting effectiveness, while acute problems may just take one or two treatments. It is reported that AcuScen proves effective in 80% of all cases, of which full recovery occurs in two-thirds of them, with significant healing in the remainder.

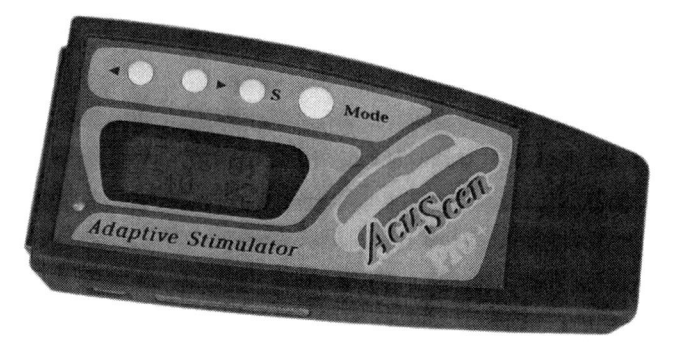

This is a photo of the AcuScen Pro device. The display shows the energetic response from the patient and gives the user the opportunity to adjust the AcuScen signal to match what the energy system needs to get Ki flowing. Photo courtesy of Mikhail Teppone, M.D.

    I consider AcuScen/SCENAR one of my most amazing and effective non-invasive energy medicine discoveries. The healing possibilities are incredible and no drugs or surgery is required. Think out-of-the-box and contact an AcuScen practitioner near you or contact Dr. Mikhail Teppone.

These statements have not been evaluated by the Food and Drug Administration. This product is not intended to diagnose, treat, cure, or prevent disease

Chapter 9
Bio-Energetic Screening
(Bio-Resonance Therapy)

Bio-Energetic Screening (BES) provides yet more proof that our life force energy, Ki, is manageable by us. We can take active steps to balance and clear this energy in order to improve every aspect of our health and life. This amazing technology has actually been granted United States FDA approval for certain therapeutic applications, particularly in the area of allergy diagnosis

BES is placed in this chapter on energetic healing, but it could just as well have been placed in the section on Healing Diets, Vitamins, Herbs, Allergies, and Electro Magnetic Frequencies, because this technology deals with all of these and more: health screening, allergy determination, nutritional supplement determination, and broader diagnosis of wellness.

BES is a receiver for the electromagnetic signals that our bodies emit. Everything in this Universe emits a unique energetic frequency or footprint.

The unit takes your energetic reading and produces a homeopathic with the healing energies that may be useful to your body. The BES is a form of biofeedback that measures the bio-energetic system of the body, using the same Ki energy that traditional Chinese medicine has recognized and worked with for centuries. Diagnosis and treatment of diseases can be accomplished by stimulating these energy centers just as we have seen in other energetic medicine. Like the others, this treatment is totally non-invasive. The Asyra is like body radar. It shows precisely where the enemy (bacteria, parasites, virus's emotional distress, etc.) is by recognizing its unique bio electronic signal. Once the signal is received by the Asyra, it then provides a homeopathic energetic remedy and a list of naturopathic nutritionals to treat the specific ailments.

This technology was developed in the 1950s when German physician Voll refined a diagnostic technique using the acupuncture potent points to accurately pinpoint specific weaknesses in a patient's body according to Voll. This technique, called Electro Acupuncture, has been in widespread use since its discovery. Dr. Voll's EAV invention has been continually upgraded to the present day with the latest in computer technology, software, and a broad range of diagnostic filters that recognize disease frequencies as they are broadcast by the body.

The EAV and related BES technologies have been in use for years in conven¬tional medicine for the successful diagnosis and treatment of allergies. This isn't witch craft, but tried and true medicine, with FDA approval (in some areas). Here's an example of another healing technique that passed me by for decades. I guess I wasn't ready for it until now? Most of these things are found when you're ready for them.

My Experience

In my continuing quest to understand what makes me "tick", and more specifically identify the vitamins and minerals I need to improve my health, I enlisted the services of a Naturopath here in Austin. She had just taken delivery of a brand new, state-of-the-art BES unit and offered to try it out on me.

The BES system used was called Asyra, which means "the healer who uses resosnance analysis." After being activated, the unit started reading the electrical signals emanating from the palms of my hands and generating a diagnosis at lightning speed. Data flashed across the screen as my bio electronic frequencies were broadcast into the unit, analyzed, and stored. Very Star Wars!

Bio-Energetic Screening

This particular model, the Asyra AT3™, was just released in 2007.[1] This unit has a breakthrough upgrade that reduces hours and hours of diagnostic work into a 10 minute session. With the older Asyra models, the operator would have to go around your body, pressing on specific potent points with a probe while the unit measured your body's energetic response. The readings were recorded and output available at the end of the multi-hour session. The time savings, ease of use features, and reductions in operator-error make the Asyra AT3™ a more practical and effective healing tool. Additionally, it has brought the cost of use way down and dramatically improved the productivity of the healer. (I don't know if I would have been able to sit through a tedious multi-hour treatment with last year's model or been able to afford to pay the bill since the treatment isn't covered by medical insurance.)[2]

Once the unit was turned on it started taking energetic readings and measuring my body's capacitive reaction. It picked up frequencies from my body that related to specific issues like allergies, vitamin deficiencies, viruses, parasites, emotional distress, and diseases that emitted specific, measureable frequencies recognized by the Asyra AT3™. (The filter or frequency database gets continually updated by naturopaths and other healing practitioners.) The unit is picking up "distress signals" and recording them in the computer. It "knows" what a healthy organ or cell frequency looks like versus an unhealthy frequency. As with standard software programs, enhancements and upgrades are constantly being added.

My personal Asyra AT3™ bio-electronic analysis indicated multiple disease signatures, allergies, parasites, and some emotional stress that were being broadcast as an electronic signal from my body, bringing to light and confirming something that I had known for years; disease and sickness are layered phenomena. Like an onion, the more layers you peel away, the more disease-creating energies

---

[1] *Asyra AT3™ is a trademark of Gtech™ LLC.*
[2] *I received Asyra AT3™ treatments at Awakening Health, Austin Texas, Meridian Grace, ND 2007–2008*

are exposed. This layering phenomenon is also present in emotional issues and in the information that is stored in the subconscious.

So although you may think that you have identified the source of your sickness, very often times it is just a surface issue that is concealing several others that, when resolved, will make you totally healthy. For the Asyra AT3™ therapy to work effectively, you need to have readings taken over a period of months so that each layer can be exposed. This is how you arrive at the "core issues."

Sicknesses from early childhood and, in my case, early adult years that were "treated," never really went away. You may think that you were "cured," but very often the sickness hasn't left your body. It gets weakened and then hibernates deep in your tissues or organs where it may emerge later when you least suspect it or it may remain dormant for your entire life. When they say that XYZ bacteria or virus leads to XYZ cancer, it is usually because you've been carrying these things and they were quietly multiplying and growing in strength deep within your body without your knowledge. You don't feel anything until the cancer cells grow in sufficient size to cause discomfort and disease.

I have learned that the liver, spleen, adrenal glands, thyroid, heart, kidneys, lymph, and other areas of the body can harbor diseases for years in semi-dormant states. They are waiting for your immune system to weaken due to toxicity, stress, fatigue, emotional upset, trauma, or any number of other disease triggering events or conditions. At the core they are mental or emotional ultimately manifesting themselves in the physical form.

The Asyra AT3™ is like body radar. It shows precisely where the enemy (bac¬teria, parasites, viruses emotional distress, etc.) are by recognizing their unique bio electronic signal. Once the signal is received by the Asyra AT3™, it then outputs a homeopathic energetic solution and a list of naturopathic nutritionals to treat the specific ailments.

To me this is mind blowing stuff. But I get off on this kind of thing. I like "knowing". I've gotten over my early belief that "ignorance is bliss" when it comes to diseases. I want to know early and head the disease off at the pass, if I can.

If you're interested in this type of diagnosis and treatment, contact Asyra AT3™. They can direct you to a trained practitioner in your area.

These are some of the ailments that have been treted with bioenergetic screening:

Arthritis	**Hyperactivity**
Asthma	**Irritable Bowel**
Candida	**Menopause**
Eczema	**Migraine**
Energy levels	**Prostate**
Environmental Sensitivity	**Thyroid**
Food and Nutrition	**Toxicity**
Hormone Levels	

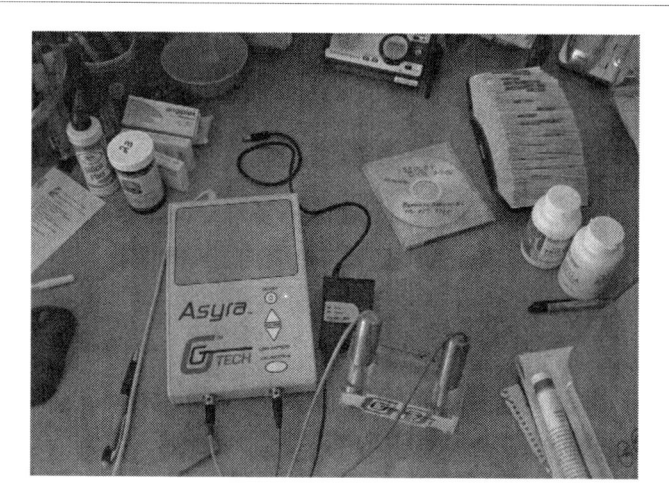

This is the Asyra AT3™ that was used on me for bio-energetic screening. It is manufactured by Gtech™. The brass handles are held in each hand while the Asyra AT3™ unit takes readings of your body's electromagnetic frequencies.

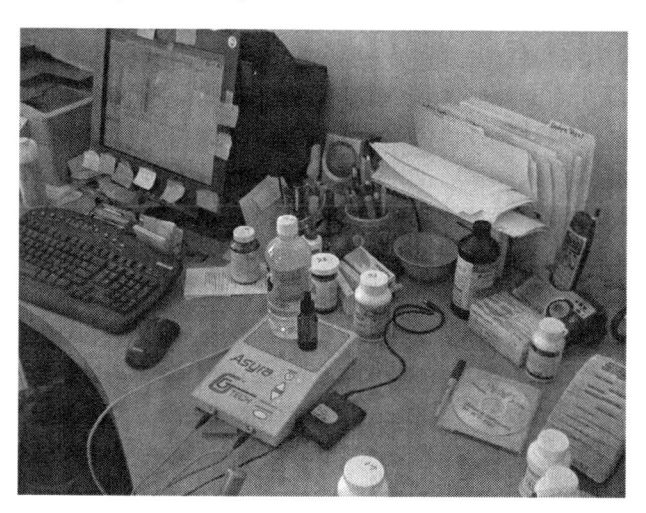

The Asyra AT3™ is connected to a computer that houses special software. You receive a report on your condition and a homeopathic at the end of a session. In this photo, two nutritionals are being evaluated for compatibility with my present condition as evaluated by the Asyra AT3™ assessment that I just completed.

Chapter 10
Emotional Freedom Technique
Self Administered Acupressure

Emotional Freedom Technique (EMT) was developed by Gary Craig, a Stanford-trained engineer.[3]

I have, over the years, been treated with acupuncture, light acupuncture, acupressure, reiki, and shiatsu massage for allergies and upper respiratory ailments. I was very familiar with the benefits of stimulating the energy channels of the meridians and using potent points in the body to trigger healing used in traditional Chinese medicine. The concept of using these same potent points and meridians for emotional healing intrigued me, so I immediately recognized the connection and grasped the tremendous potential benefits of EFT. The basic tenet of this therapy (like other energy-focused therapies) is getting you to deal with unresolved angers, fears, and traumas that have stored in our mind and bodies that later show up as disease or emotional issues and interfere with living a peaceful life.

Craig merged rapid eye movement, acupressure, creative visualization, and affirmations into a self-treatment therapy that anyone can use on anything. He encouraged his patients to explore the possibilities because everything in your body involves the movement or blockage of energy.

Very similar to acupuncture and acupressure, it uses the 14 meridians, that were mapped by the Chinese thousands of years ago, to release energy blocks. The difference is that the EFT user is

---

3   www.emofree.com, This is Gary Craig's website on EFT

focusing on a specific problem, tapping potent points, and verbally reciting specific commands about the problem in question. This process is shown to break up energy blockages in the body, allowing Ki, or electrical energy, to flow freely. The free flow of energy allows health to be restored and dislodges embedded negative emotions.

I think this has huge potential in treating our soldiers coming back from Iraq and Afghanistan. It should also be explored in our prison system, since most violence is rooted in early childhood trauma, neglect, and abuse. Releasing these blockages may provide relief for many deep-rooted conditions.

EFT has been shown to work on: allergies, asthma, colds, high blood pressure, muscle sprains, fears, phobias and anxieties.

Finally, Craig recommends that people try it on everything since it's easy and, you never know, it may work! It certainly can't hurt you.

My Experience

Craig has a series of DVDs that are totally unrehearsed healing sessions with a broad spectrum of people. I recommend that, if you are considering EFT, you see that it truly works before trying it. There are people with arthritis, asthma, post-traumatic stress disorder, fear of heights, and almost any malady you can think of gaining benefits from EFT. These live case studies were what convinced me that this works.

Gary Craig's website (http://www.emofree.com) and download his FREE instructions on how to perform EFT on yourself.

I've tried EFT on numerous occasions and I think it works on me. Since I multi-task on my health care using a combination of exercise, nutrition, meditation, along with EFT, it's hard to know for sure what exact role it has played in my recovery from any one thing. Maybe nothing. The same can be said for acupuncture. I'm confident it contributed to healing, but I needed other things in conjunction with it to heal myself. This is actually quite common.

Trying this out is a no-brainer; energy medicine, in a simple, easy, and free form. If you don't get the results you are seeking, enlist the services of a certified EFT practitioner. There are nuances to the setup, clearly articulating the problem you want to resolve, and rating your EFT responses of the scale of 1 to 10. Check it out. It's worth a try.

Chapter 11
Massage Therapies

Massage is a relaxing and therapeutic way to get energy flowing through your body. It can also push toxins trapped or stagnating in your tissues out into your circulatory system and, ultimately, out of your body.

Massage is the practice of stroking and applying pressure to the soft tissues of the body, including muscles, tendons, connective tissue, and joints. Effective massage improves circulation, heals injury, relieves stress and tension, and aids in the elimination of waste products. The most well known massage movements are per¬cussion (tapotement), kneading (petrissage), and stroking or gliding (effleurage). There are over 80 different massage techniques, of which I have experienced 5.4

My Experience

Massage is a great method to relieve stress, relax tight muscles, and drain the lymphatic system of toxins (lactic acid, uric acid, and other waste products). Massage therapists claim that it can relieve sinus problems, breathing disorders, digestive problems, circulatory problems, migraines, back problems, tension and stress.

The massage practitioners that I have used typically included a combination of techniques in their practice: Deep tissue, Swedish, Reiki, Reflexology, and Shiatsu. Each technique delivers a different health-giving benefit. The Author has tried all of the massage therapies listed here.

Deep Tissue Massage

As the name suggests, this technique focuses on the deeper layers of muscle tissue. Slow strokes and deep finger pressure are focused in areas where muscle tension has built up. Pressure is applied along and across the muscle fibers. It can be slightly painful, but is effective in loosening muscles, improving circulation, and helping eliminate toxins from the muscle tissue. A massage therapist will usually ask you how the pressure feels and back off if you are uncomfortable.

I usually work through the heavy pressure and discomfort as I feel the end result is worth a little pain. After a deep tissue massage,I feel euphoric, albeit slightly light headed, a little sore and drowsy. Following a session I drink at least a quart of spring water. My sleep is usually deep and uninterrupted.

Swedish Massage

This technique, developed in the 1700s by a Swedish doctor Per Henrik Ling, focuses on the deeper muscles and bones. Rubbing in the same direction as the flow of blood returning to the heart, Swedish massage uses long strokes, kneading movement, vibration, tapping, along with bending and stretching the limbs.

I have found that a straight Swedish massage is less strenuous than the deep tissue massage because less pressure is applied and the type of techniques employed.

Reflexology

Reflexology was brought to this country by Chinese immigrants. It focuses on the feet and hands, with the practitioner applying pressure using the thumb and hands. As in traditional Chinese medicine, there are neural connections between the feet and hands that correspond to the major organs in the body. Gently rubbing focused areas of the feet and hands can clear out congestion and restore normal health.

During reflexology I have gotten sensations in my stomach and liver area that directly corresponded to the area being manipulated during the session. Having felt this connection first-hand, I really believe that it works.

Reiki

Originated in Tibet, Reiki has been practiced in that region for thousands of years. The focus is on channeling the Universal Life Force, or Chi, to heal ailments.

Reiki practitioners use their hands to channel energy into the subject's body for healing. I had Reiki applied by a practitioner in conjunction with other techniques. As a result, I could not specifically detect its effects in treating a particular ailment, so I cannot personally say how it works. However, I've heard from many people that it is very healing.

Shiatsu

Coming from Japan, Shiatsu is a technique whereby finger pressure is applied across areas of energy lines or meridians (like acupuncture), to promote good health by stimulating the body's energy flow or Ki.

I suggest that, if you have not tried massage, find a licensed, certified practitioner. Use it to promote energy flow in your body. All of the great athletes of our time; Formula One drivers, gymnasts, figure skaters, weight lifters, cyclists, baseball players, soccer players, and football players regularly use massage therapy to help heal and rejuvenate their bodies.

Chapter 12
Light and Color Therapy

"Light is present in every cell of our bodies. It is extremely faint- the intensity of a candle flame seen at 25 kilometers-radiation from living cells...the purpose is intra and intercellular regulation and communication."

— Dr. Fritz-Albert Popp

Did it ever occur to you all kinds of illnesses can be cured with light and color? It never occurred to me until I started writing this book and began to discover an incredible body of work about these methods of healing. There are some breakthrough therapies that use light and color. You will learn about some of the healing secrets of light and color in this chapter.

The readily recognized and widely used area of light treatment is laser technology. (I am not covering the use of lasers here, but they have been used in the following areas: eye site correction, skin treatment, microsurgery, and orthopedic surgery.) The light therapy I will discuss, like all of the other therapies in this book, requires no incisions or burning of tissues to be effective.

Light is a fundamental building block of nature. It is in everything and, as I have learned, can be used to fix an incredible number of ailments and imbalances in our bodies. These discoveries of light, color, and crystals are new to me, but their origins date back to the dawn of civilization. Why haven't I seen or heard about this energy before? I think we learned the answer to this question in Chapter 3.

The revelation for me was that Light and Color therapies have been in pretty widely used for decades. When you are brought up believing medicine comes in a pill box or bottle, it is hard to accept that a beam of light or a color or a crystal could be emitting healing energy. When was the last time that you made a visit to your light doctor (Syntonic Optometrist)? If you are like me, the answer is never. The healing powers of light and color are not well known to the broad population; at least not in my travels. These relatively unknown therapies can offer truly miraculous results for a wide diversity of conditions. Here are a few examples of light therapy:

Therapy	Treatment
Light and Color	An incredible number of healing modalities involve the use of light and color. Light and Color therapies are available to treat cancer, depression, anxiety, sleep disorders, malnutrition, post-traumatic stress disorder, Seasonal Affective Disorder (SAD), jet lag, dyslexia, learning ability, blood quality, and AIDS. We are "light beings," therefore it stands to reason that light and color should be key sources for healing.
Rife Beam	Rife beam ray In the 1920's, a man named Royal Rife discovered, through the use of a special microscope and lighting, that each microorganism has its own unique light and resonant frequency. He further determined that you could tune into this resonant frequency, manipulate it and destroy it. By using specially tuned light, he was able to destroy bacteria and viruses. He used this knowledge in cancer research at the University of Southern California where he was able to isolate organisms from cancer tissue and destroy them and heal the cancer. His success rate was 90% using the rife beam.[1]

Therapy	Treatment
Lumatron Light Simulator	Developed by Dr. John Downing. Used by: Chiropractors for adjustments to the autonomic nervous system. Optometrists for enlarging visual fields and rehab of the neuro visual system. Psychiatrists: for alleviation of mental and emotional problems, like Post-Traumatic Stress Disorder. Seasonal Affective Disorder, anxiety, depression, sleep disorders, speech, light sensitivity, panic attacks, and repressed memories. Naturopaths: for a full range of physiological imbalances.[2]
Photphrin	Photphrin Photodynamic therapy (PDT) is a treatment regimen developed by Dr. Thomas Dougherty, at the Roswell Park Institute in Buffalo, NY. He discovered that intravenously injected photosensitive chemicals (DHE or photofrin) accumulate in cancer cells, which can then be identified under ultraviolet light. (The cancer cells give off a red glow. Most healthy cells do not.) Dougherty then directed red light at the cancer cells destroying them with no adverse effect on the surrounding healthy cells[3] Photofrin can locate cancer cells and at the same time destroy them. By 1992, over 3,000 cancer patients, with a wide variety of malignant tumors, had been treated using PDT. Success Rate: 70–80% after only one treatment. (Chart continued on next page)

[1] Cooper, Primrose. *The Healing Power of Light*. York Beach, ME: Weiser Books, Inc., 2001

Therapy	Treatment
Photphrin	Photofrin can locate cancer cells and at the same time destroy them. By 1992, over 3,000 cancer patients, with a wide variety of malignant tumors, had been treated using PDT.Success Rate: 70–80% after only one treatment. Success depends in large measure on the ability to get light to the tumor. Large, deeply embedded tumors and those that have spread (metastasized) are not as easily treated due to their inaccessibility to light exposure. [National Cancer Institute] Side Effects: light sensitivity, skin sensitivity

Like plants, humans need full spectrum sunlight, that is sunlight with all of the colors you see in a rainbow, to nourish our bodies and minds. There are processes somewhat similar to photosynthesis in plants that take place when our bodies are exposed to sunlight or full spectrum light[8]. The most obvious is the production of the hormone calcitrol, or vitamin D, by the kidneys. This is a key agent in calcium absorption and cancer fighting properties. The production of melatonin in the pineal gland, located in the brain, is influenced by the light that comes through our eyes. Melatonin regulates our sleep cycle and biological clock. Light affects the presence of life itself. It governs the rate of growth of cells and tissue. Light impacts reproductive functions, heredity, bodily chemical processes, and learning ability.

When light is broken down it is composed of colors that perform different functions in the body and correspond to different areas. The pallet includes:

---

2   Breiling, Brian et al. *Light Years Ahead.* Berkeley,Ca:Light Years Ahead Publishing. 1996. Pages 227–231.

3   Breiling, Brian et al. *Light Years Ahead.* Berkeley,Ca:Light Years Ahead Publishing. 1996. Pages 112–113.

Ruby, Red, Red/Orange, Orange, Yellow, Yellow/Green, Blue/Green, Blue, Indigo and Violet

You can add turquoise and other shades of these colors, but these are the basic colors of the light spectrum that comes from sunlight.

The energy from sun and light permeates all things. The individual colors in light correspond to different parts of our anatomy and energy centers or chakras. Energy flows in and out of our body through the chakras. When you are sick or emotionally out of sorts, chances are that your color energy is out of balance and needs supplementation.

Basic color chart[9]:

Color	Chakra	Gland	Body Area	Gem(s)
Violet/White	Crown	Pineal	Top of Head	Amethyst/ Clear Quartz
Indigo	"Third Eye"	Pituitary	Forehead	Lapis
Blue	Throat	Thyroid	Throat	Sodalite
Green	Heart	Thymus	Center of Chest	Jade/ Moldavite
Yellow	Solar Plexus	Spleen	Under Diaphram	Topaz/ Citrine
Orange	Sacrum	Ovaries/ Testes	Lower Abdomen	Amber/ Carnelian
Red	Root	Adrenals	Base of Spine	Garnet/Ruby

To understand the medical and scientific basis of the healing power of light and color I recommend reading *Light Years Ahead*, a compilation of presentations by some of the best medical authorities on the subject, and *Light Medicine of the Future* by Dr. Jacob Liberman. There is no sense in me repaving this cow path when you

---

4   Dispenza, Joseph. *Live Better Longer: The Parcells Center 7-Step Plan for Health and Longevity.* Lincoln, Nebr: iUniverse.com, Inc. 2000

5   Breiling, Brian et al. *Light Years Ahead.* Berkeley,Ca:Light Years Ahead Publishing. 1996. Page 240

can learn directly from real experts about the miraculous qualities of light healing.

Areas of healing: Dyslexia, depression, epilepsy, Seasonal Affective Disorder, premenstrual syndrome, insomnia, cancer, multiple sclerosis.

At its most basic level, color and light impact the sympathetic nervous system and the para-sympathetic nervous system. The sympathetic nervous system is the stress-producing part of the nervous system and activates the thyroid, adrenal medulla, pituitary, testes, and muscles. The parasympathetic nervous system is opposite and activates the parathyroids, adrenal cortex, digestive tract, liver, pancreas, and spleen.

Light works like Chi in traditional Chinese medicine in that, if it is balanced and flowing at the right level, you are healthy. If it gets depleted or blocked, it causes disease. The depletion of light can be seen by Kirlian photography of the aura. A person who is diseased or stressed-out will exhibit a non-symmetrical, distorted red aura or have patches of aura that are completely missing.

There is another theory about how light affects people. It is said that at the time a specific emotion is triggered in the brain, light is sent through the body, ultimately finding a resting place in tissues and organs. Trauma can also be transmitted through the body in the form of light and find a resting place in an organ. The trauma is always there unless a pro-active treatment of light is used to ferret it out of the system. It's just like freeing a Chi block through acupuncture administered to the potent point corresponding to the blocked area of the body.

With professionally administered light or crystal therapy you can restore the symmetry and color to the aura. Violet and white around the crown chakra are symptomatic of a healthy aura.

My Experience

When I had a Kirlian photograph taken, my aura was red and orange, a sign of a type A, aggressive personality. I think I had too much coffee before the photo was taken!

I am convinced that light and color possess incredible healing power and will become the leading edge of therapy in the future. The use of light for healing dates back to ancient Egypt, China, and India.

I first I read about the potential of light and color in Dr. Lieberman's book, then in Joseph Dispenza's excellent book *Live Better Longer*, which describes how Dr. Hazel Parcels used color therapy with many of her patients.

Here is a list of the things I've tried, starting with the most obvious and basic, and then moving into the more unusual. Many of these were adopted from reading *Live Better Longer*, where there is a comprehensive list of therapies.

Sunbathing

15 to 30 minutes a day to produce vitamin D (calcitriol) in the body, 2 to 3 times a week, preferably before 11:00 am or after 3:00 pm, when the sun's rays are less intense.

Go easy on the sunscreen as most commercial brands (ironically) are carcinogenic. If you have fair skin, get your exposure very early in the morning or late afternoon. Sit in a slightly shaded area or in indirect sunlight. Sun light is good. Contrary to the BS you've been taught, the sun is good for you. You need the sun; just not too much.

Full Spectrum Light

Full spectrum light bulbs are used in my home and office to improve our moods, prevent SAD, kill airborne bacteria, and learning and information retention. Although not as good the sun, it also helps in the production of vitamin D, Full spectrum lights are used in some hospitals to prevent the spread of airborne germs like staph.

Rainbow Diet

Eat raw and cooked vegetables that correspond to the sun's spectrum to replenish color in the body. Mix red radishes/beets/tomatoes, purple eggplant, yellow squash, green broccoli/spinach/collards, orange peppers/carrots, and any other colors that you can find, into a salad or stir fry to create a rainbow meal. This is just one way to absorb the colors of the rainbow.

Whether you buy into the this color business or not, these colored vegetables are a great source of antioxidants, like cartenoid licopene (tomatoes) and beta-carotene (carrots) that help fight certain cancers.

Sun Water

Place a bottle of water into direct sunlight for at least 30 minutes. The sun purifies the water and energizes it.[10]

Rainbow Water

Take a glass of distilled or spring water and place it in direct sunlight with a glass prism on top. The prism will refract the sun's rays into the seven component colors of sunlight which are then absorbed by the water. Wait 10 plus minutes before drinking the color energized water. Dr. Hazel Parcells claimed that distilled water works best, as it is a sponge for anything into which it comes into contact.

Distilled water is acidic so I usually use filtered tap water or bottled spring water. I like this because you get all of the colors in one glass of water.

---

6   Dispenza, Joseph. *Live Better Longer: The Parcells Center 7-Step Plan for Health and Longevity.* Lincoln, Nebr: iUniverse.com, Inc. 2000. Pages 136–137.

7   Dispenza, Joseph. *Live Better Longer: The Parcells Center 7-Step Plan for Health and Longevity.* Lincoln, Nebr: iUniverse.com, Inc. 2000. Pages 136–137.

Color Water

Place a colored cathedral glass over a glass of water in the sunlight. When you drink the water the color is passed on to you. Each individual color has a specific effect on the mind and body. I use two colors on a regular basis.

Blue water: Calms the nerves, lowers the pulse, and helps with sleep

Yellow water: Aids in digestion

I drink a lot of lemon juice mixed with water since the color yellow lifts the mood. Lemon juice brightens the spirits and has an alkalizing effect on the body. It is an excellent internal cleansing agent.

Do these really work? I think they do, but I have no proof. I use color water for the fun of it and because it is simple to do. In the best case, I am getting color necessary for life into my body. In the worst case, they don't work, but I am still getting a refreshing glass of water. There is no harm and a potentially big upside to color water.

Here's a guide that Dr. Parcells assembled for color therapy:

Dr. Parcell's application and uses of colors[1].

Color	Application/Effect
Violet	Heart, nerve, blood pressure depressant. Works with the spleen to increase white blood cell count.
Blue	Slows fast pulse. Pain reliever, reduces body temperature, and is a heart sedative.
Green	Antiseptic, stimulates pituitary gland. Work with lymphatic system. Encourages absorption of medication.
Yellow	Laxative, digestion aid, and reduces swelling.

Color	Application/Effect
Orange	Asthma, respiratory issues, spasms, digestion, ulcers, thyroid function, oxygen carrier to the lungs.
Red	Excites, hemoglobin builder, works through liver and mucous membranes.
Indigo	Sedative stops hemorrhaging, overactive thyroid gland, high blood pressure, emotional trauma.

Color Acupuncture (The Bioptron™ light therapy)

After reading about the phenomenal healing results in the book Light Years Ahead, I had to try light therapy for myself at home. I researched the cheapest and simplest products and decided to purchase a Bioptron™ color light therapy set from Bipotron AG, Monchalytorf, Switzerland.

Bioptron™ AG has taken research information from the Zurich-based Institute for Bioinformation regarding life regeneration patterns in plants, precious stones, minerals, and trace elements, and incorporated it into its own sophisticated color therapy system. The technology is used to treat the body with color and light information. (Check out www.bioptron.com for details.)[2]

The treatment areas on the body are the same as those used for acupuncture. Light is directed a few inches from potent points on the skin at various locations around the body in specific sequences and for specific time durations. Colored light is used in conjunction with scented plant-based creams.

Bioptron is like a high tech spa treatment for the home with intelligence that is broadcast into your body and tissues. Don't ask me how it works. The technical details are closely guarded secrets and are not available from Bioptron. They do claim to have been used to successfully treat many people for sleep disorders, energy/vitality, skin disorders, digestion, purging, memory, concentration, motivation, fear, and lack of drive.

The kit I bought included a polarized light, red, orange, yellow, green, blue, and violet colored glass filters (impregnated with bioinformation), and plant-based scented creams. The impregnation with bioinformation is the piece that I don't understand, but I guess it's some secret of nature that they discovered and encoded into glass. (sacred geometric shapes or patterns? My guess.)

My Experience

I have tried three of the twelve Bioptron™ therapies: Inner balance, Vital spark, and supporting resistance. These treatments entail applying scented aromatic cream to the treatment area (various acupuncture potent points) and then holding the colored, polarized light 2 inches from the location, for a variety of time durations, according to the treatment regimen.

Since I was not suffering from any specific sickness when I bought my Bioptron kit, it was difficult to determine if this light therapy worked. I think this is really cool and, after reading books and the Bioptron instruction manual, I am convinced, at an intuitive level, that this therapy, driven by light, color, and bioinformation works. I just can't tell you how. There was no clear, obvious health benefit to report from these self-administered treatments. I can report being fully relaxed and my sleep seemed to be more restful, but these are subjective opinions, not hard facts.

My take away from this experience is that it is best to go to a professional light therapy practitioner who has years of clinical experience with a variety of patients. I purchased a home wellness kit that I plan to use from time to time for health maintenance and not any particular illness. I accept the opinion that the body needs light and color and that the Bioptron™ is a very efficient way to get deep, penetrating light into the body. Naturally this light therapy is not sanctioned or approved by the United States Federal

---

8   Bioptron AG, Editors, *Bioptron Colour Therapy Basics*, Monchaltorf, Switzerland, 1998.

Drug Administration, but neither are a majority of homeopathic, naturopathic treatments.

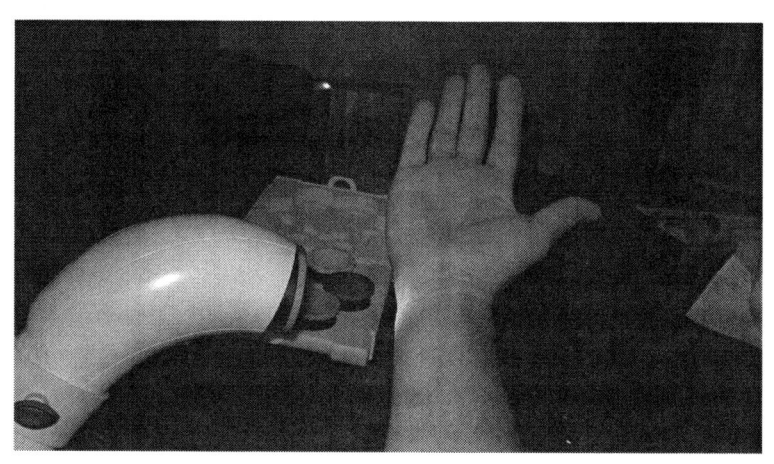

This is color therapy using the Bioptron™ polar light, focusing on a specific potent point this is one of many ways to move energy in your body and to clear energetic blockages.

"We are born of light, we live in light, and we die in light. We are made of light. Everything is made of light. Science has come to this understanding by a very long route."
    — Ohso in Scriptures in *Silence and Sermons in Stones*

Chapter 13
Crystals and Gems

Crystals and gems are probably the oldest tools employed by man for healing that combine light, color, and other resonant, healing frequencies. All of the ancient cultures attributed healing properties to crystals and gems and used them as healing remedies and religious symbols, jewelry, art, and currency.

In Ayurvedic medicine, gems are crushed into a fine powder for specific remedies and consumed orally. In homeopathy they are made into liquid essences.

To start my investigation on gem healing I obtained a book that I thought would provide objective and scientific proof that crystals really do have healing power. I wanted empirical, fact-based evidence that there was some merit to using crystals for healing purposes. I was told that the authoritative source for this information is *Crystal Power, Crystal Healing* by Michael Gienger.

The author has a degree in chemistry and mineralogy from the University of Stuttgart in Germany. He got deeply into crystals after curing himself from severe sinusitis (severe sinus infection) with an emerald, after antibiotics and other conventional drugs failed to provide relief. Based on this experience, he decided to dedicate his life to the study of the healing properties of minerals using science as a basis for his research. According to Gienger,

> "The healing properties of minerals and all other types of stone can be traced back to the manner of their origin, their inner structure, their mineral elements and their

colors. These four principles can be described separately and in the case of each individual stone, can be combined to form an individual portrait of its healing characteristics."[1] Basically, at a very basic level, we humans are physically attracted to stones and derive healing power from their resonance that is needed to balance our system. Since we all originate from Mother Earth, we have a kinship with all of her basic elements. Being made of earth elements, it stands to reason that we are attracted to, resonate with, derive nutrition from, and can heal our bodies with stones and their base elements."

Take a look at a list of elements that can be found in small traces in your body: Copper, silver, gold, nickel, zinc, silicon, titanium, calcium, vanadium, manganese, iron, selenium, sodium, sulphur, and potassium.

An interesting story that confirms this attraction, and may apply to all of us, is a discovery Gienger made about the earth below our feet. After studying the geology of his birthplace and seven different residences up to that time, he discovered that the first five had the same types of soil and rock. "Was this a coincidence?" he asked, or is there a natural, biological attraction that we have to subterranean rock and soil? He believed that this was no coincidence, but a real attraction; a natural magnetism exists between us and our home soil and earth. At some very deep, unconscious level, we have a connection with geology, Mother Earth or "Gaia." You oftentimes hear refugees or immigrants say that they want to return to their soil or want to be buried in ground from the town where they were born. I think there is more than just sentimentality at work here. There is some physical and spiritual attraction.

So how do crystals work in healing? Again I quote Gienger:

---

[1] Gienger, Michael. *Crystal Power, Crystal Healing.* New York: Sterling Publishing Co., 1998. Page 13.

"What form does the communication between stone and human take place? How and through what means do minerals unleash their healing effects? How can a piece of matter influence a living organism?'

The healing effect of a crystal becomes more easily understandable if we put aside the notion that the limits of our being are identical with the limits of our physical bodies. This notion is definitely a fallacy. Even in physics it has been known for well over a hundred years that everybody, every organism, every "material object", be it a stone, a plant, or a plastic bucket, possesses what is referred to variously as an "emanation" or aura. Many physical and all chemical processes involve the absorption and emanation of radiation, which means that whatever takes place, heat, light, or another form of electromagnetic radiation is either absorbed or heat, light or another form of electromagnetic radiation is released. We are all constant receivers and transmitters of radiation.[2]

Stones, minerals, and crystals also possess radiating properties. Their radiation results from the transformation of absorbed light, lying mainly in the infrared region and only to a very small degree in the visible and microwave regions of the spectrum. But in spite of their lesser quantity, the latter are of great importance. Infrared radiation is absorbed by the outermost layers of the skin into the body, which is why we feel it as heat. Microwaves however, penetrate the entire organism, so in principle, reach all tissues and organs."[3]

This is exactly what is taking place between stones and humans. Stones, too, emit radiation and, being extremely durable and

---

[2] Gienger, Michael. *Crystal Power, Crystal Healing.* New York: Sterling Publishing Co., 1998. page 147

[3] Gienger, Michael. *Crystal Power, Crystal Healing.* New York: Sterling Publishing Co., 1998. p 148

permanent, emit the same information in a very constant way. They can be compared to radio transmitters that constantly broadcast the same program over and over. Every stone or crystal has its own specific light or, put another way, specific radiation, that naturally influences organisms. When contact is made between crystals and our bodies, the absorbed light influences the light communication between the cells causing certain reactions.

Healing crystals fit into a category of treatments called "information therapy" which includes homeopathy and aromatherapy. It is not a chemical reaction that does the healing (like medicines or herbs), but the "information" emitted by them. This is the best explanation I can find. Gienger goes into some of the specific chemical and physical properties of crystals in his book which I won't cover because chemistry is not my strong suit.

My Experience

I have no doubt that crystals have healing properties. However, I have not found or encountered a crystal healing method, personally, that delivers dramatic, measureable, and consistent healing results. I've concluded that there are so many advanced and powerful, natural, energetic healing tools that are available to me, that using crystals seems like a step back into the "Stone Age." I would use AcuScen, bio-energetic screening, acupuncture, and radionics before crystals. I know that to crystal healers this sounds like some close-minded conventional medicine bigot, but I think there are devices that do what crystals are supposed to do faster, more reliably, with a higher degree of consistency; taking the guess work out of healing. If you read this and disagree, please show me an example. I'm ready to see it and believe it. So far, I haven't found one that works for me. Gienger makes a very convincing case in his book so I'm not dismissing crystal healing, I just haven't experienced it on a broad level (Himalayan salt lamps, the exception).

I find crystals aesthetically and energetically appealing In fact, I can't walk into a store that sells crystals without buying at least one. So I'm an aficionado and do believe they have incredible energy. I think their use in healing is very "hit or miss" and you need to look really hard to find an expert crystal healer.

My Experience

Himalayan Salt Crystal Lamps

By keeping salt lamps in our bedrooms, my family has experienced some minor relief from allergy discomfort. I am told that they work like this: Himalayan salt crystal lamps are negative ion generators that interact energetically and chemically with the surrounding environment. There is a chemical interaction or "transformation cycle" that takes place between the oxygen, hydrogen, sodium and chloride ions released by the crystals. I have no clue what this means, but can tell you that it works.

Another benefit that is said to be derived from negative ion generation is the absorption of positive ions generated by computers, television sets, cell phones, electric motors, and other electric appliances, in the form of electromagnetic frequencies (EMF). The resonant frequency of the salt lamp is said to neutralize these harmful high frequencies.

I have no scientific proof this works, but just in case I have a salt crystal near my computer and IP telephone in my office. I get plenty of weird looks at work and comments about this pink crystal on my desk and even a few giggles. Laughter is very healing so I guess it does work.

Pink Himalayan Sea Salt (Food Grade)

The crushed pink salt crystals that I use contain up to 82 trace minerals making them very nutritious, tasty, and energizing. I use this pink salt and sea salt instead of regular iodized salt.

Thai Crystal Deodorant Stone

Yes there is a crystal that reduces body odor and it actually works. According to the label, it is made with mineral salts.

Laying Of Stones & Chakra Clearing

There is a practice in energy medicine of laying colored gemstones on your chakras according to their corresponding colors. (Please see the preceding chakra/color chart to identify the seven chakras and stones.)

I have tried this, a couple of times, for meditation and relaxation purposes. Since I was not targeting any specific ailment, I can only say that I found it relaxing, but cannot say that I received any therapeutic benefit.

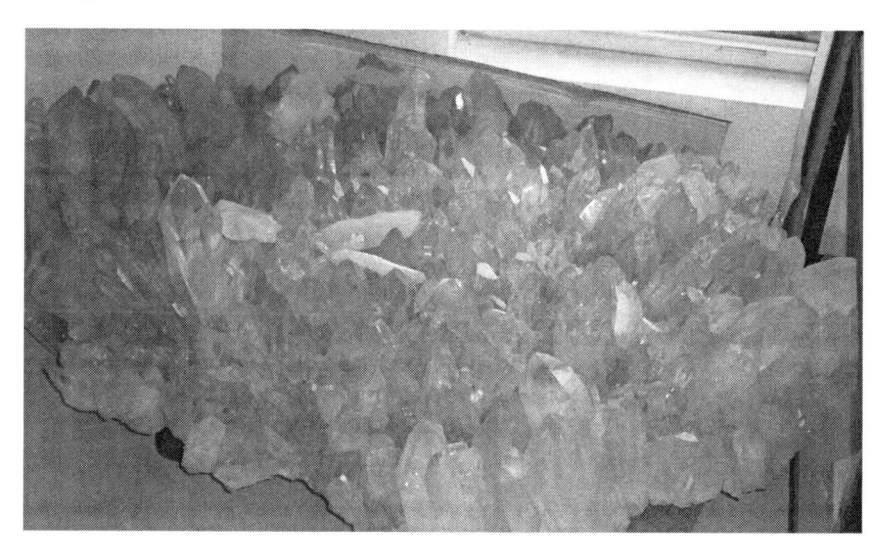

This is the largest crystal cluster that I've ever seen. This photo was taken at the Coleman Mine Warehouse. The Coleman's own the largest crystal mines in Arkansas. I went to Jessieville, Arkansas near Hots Springs in the Ozark Mountains to Coleman mines as part of the research for this book. This is a pretty magical part of the country with some of the largest crystal mines in the world and the famous hot springs. This whole area was sacred to Native Americans.

I went specifically to talk crystals with the Colemans and buy a few crystals for my modest collection. I personally have not harnessed the healing power of crystals but know it's there.

Just for fun I am listing some of the crystals that I own and the medicinal properties that are attributed to them.

Sample Crystal Healing Properties[4]

The healing properties attributed to these crystals and gems are unconfirmed (by me). They are provided here as an example of what crystal healers attribute to stones.

Crystal/Gem	Healing Properties
Calcite	Growth of cells, bones, community, physical development, distinction/ discrimination, heart, heart rhythm, immune system, memory, metabolism, overcoming scurvy, skin, success, tissues, tumors, wound healing
Rose quartz	Certainty, fertility, heart, heart rhythm, helpfulness, love, meditation, needs, open-mindedness and receptiveness, radiation, self love, sensitivity, sexual organs, sexuality, tenderness, tissues, sense of well being, worries/carefree
Amethyst	Action, addiction, clearness, concentration, confrontation (readiness) diarrhea, dreams, gentleness, head/ headaches, holding back, honesty/sincerity, injuries, inspiration, intestines, intoxication, intuition
Smokey Quartz	Back problems, concentration, cramps, exertion, fungal infections, pain, protection, radiation, realism, relaxation, resistance of power, stress, suffering, tenseness, thinking clearly, work energy

---

4 Gienger, Michael. *Crystal Power, Crystal Healing.* New York: Sterling Publishing Co., 1998 Pages 404-114.

Crystal/Gem	Healing Properties
Malachite	Adventure, brain, confrontation, consciousness, cramps, creativity, fulfill-ment, determination, detoxification, new experiences, feelings, suppression, images, inhibitions, affirming, memory, moods, needs, observation, mental pain, pleasure, perception, shyness, tissue (connective), understanding
Garnet(s)	Action, almondine, beginnings (new), behavioral patterns, arthritis, (energy blocks, blood formation (andradite), blood quality, bodily fluids, bones (melanite), charisma (pyrope), community, confidence, conversion, courage, creativity, depression (spessartite), difficulties, distinction/discrimination, enthusiasm (uvarovite), fever (uvarovite), kidneys, metabolism, pleasure, regeneration, self confidence, sexuality, skin, stamina, taboos, wholeness, work energy, and wound healing
Rock Crystal	Realizing abilities, brain, clairvoyance, clarity, clearness, feelings of coldness, spiritual development, diarrhea, increasing effect, empathy, fever, glands, ability to learn, overcoming limitations/boundaries, meditation, memory, spiritual nature, nausea, neutrality, pain, paralysis
Citrine	Confrontation, depression, diabetes, dynamism, new experiences, extrovertness, individuality, joie de vivre/life force, meditation, mood-lifting, stomach, suppression, logical/rational thinking, variety, understanding, warmth, prosperity
Carnelian	Quality of blood, blood vessels, community, confrontation, cycles/unfinished business, solving difficulties, emotions, small intestine, metabolism, absorption of minerals, overcoming, rheumatism, steadfastness, tissues, vitamin absorption

Crystals and Gems

Crystal/Gem	Healing Properties
Imperial Topaz	Realizing abilities, activity, appetite, charisma, exhaustion, extrovert-ness, fame, fertility, generosity, ideas/abundance of ideas, life-affirming, overcoming limitations or boundaries, metabolism, nerves/nervous system, autonomous nervous system
Boji Stones	Attentiveness, behavioral patterns, energy flow, illness (gain from/causes), illness (prophylaxis)
Fluorite	Allergies, arthritis, behavioral patterns, brain, unwillingness, consciousness, dynamism, free will/free spirit, broadening horizons, external influences, injustice, intelligence/mental grasp, inventiveness, joints, learning, ability to learn, mobility/motion, mucous membranes, tumors
Moldavite	Helps identify the source of sickness and the lessons to be learned from sickness

Note: These benefits are attributed to these gems in Gienger's book. Exactly how you apply this energy, control it, monitor it, and decide when to withdraw it is a mystery to me. I know there is an answer; I just haven't found it yet.

Chapter 14
Radionics
Sending a Remedy through the Ether

"In the quantum Universe, the energy field in which a patient exists can produce healing without any need for a spatial or temporal connection. Phenomena like distant healing—healing across great distances, or even across time are conceivable."

— Norman Shealy, MD, PhD[5]

This phenomenon of distance healing has been proven to work as evidenced by the healing work of Edgar Cayce and is recognized by some quantum physicists as a very real phenomenon. My first encounter with it was in 2006. It was initially hard for me to believe until I experienced it firsthand.

There are a handful of people in my life who I told about my radionics experience before this book went to print. This was because it sounds supernatural and I didn't want people to think I had "blown a sprocket". Not a single person I told about radionics, save one, a Reiki therapist, believed what I told them about this amazing healing tool. Several people to whom I explained radionics thought that I flipped my lid. (Being a space cadet is one thing, but most of them thought I had drifted into insanity when I told them about radionics and the long-distance healing I experienced.) However, the Reiki therapist, who moves energy every day embraces the infinite potential we have as humans to move energy, so getting her to believe in long distance healing was like having a conversation

---

5 Shealy, Norman, MD. and Dawson Church, PhD. *Soul Medicine: Awakening Your Inner Blueprint for Abundant Health and Energy.* Santa Rosa, Cal.: Elite Books, 2006. Page 16

with phone repair guy about sending voices between cell phones.

If you told people 50 years ago that everyone in the world would be walking around with a wireless device that you could speak into and send your voice across the planet, they would have committed you to an insane asylum, yet all of us use cell phones everyday and just accept that they work. We've been "dumbed" down by the mass media, government, big health care, religion, and the fast food industry to the point that we no longer accept that anything is possible in nature. If it isn't on TV or available at the local grocery store, then it doesn't exist for many of us. This ignorance is slowly changing, but based on the reception I get when talking about energy medicine, we have a long, long way to go.

Radionics is a mind-blowing energy medicine that I first experienced in Albuquerque, New Mexico. I'll discuss my experience with this "magical" healing method first, then, I will have Terry Kast explain, in her own words, the process that she teaches people. Included in her section are testimonials from multiple people who, like me, experienced the wonders of Radionics and healed some really deep illnesses.

In my treatment, Terry started out with a Q2 Energy cleanse which cleared out heavy metals and toxins prior to the healer's evaluation of me using Radethesia. It's like brushing your teeth before a dental exam. You want to start with a clean surface (body) before being examined and treated. This is also a good start to any healing process. The Radethesia evaluation, a complementary energetic evaluative tool, is often used in conjunction with Radionics.

After the Q2 cleansing, I provided a photograph of myself, along with a drop of blood for evaluation. A photo of the diagnostic pad, pendulum, and homeopathics is provided. This whole concept of reading frequencies from the body was again proven to me with the Asyra bio-resonance therapy, so I have two proof points that this concept is sound. We're all giving off frequencies whether we know it or not.

My blood was then placed on a magnetic tablet with an anatomical drawing of the human body. The healer took the pendulum in her right hand and a wooden skewer in the left hand and then pointed to different areas on the anatomical drawing. (The pendulum swings clockwise when it "sees" a positive indication of an energetic imbalance and counter-clockwise when it "sees" no indication of an energetic imbalance. Different homeopathies and remedies are held to see if they resonate with the signal coming from the diagnostic tablet that is holding the photo, blood sample and the anatomical drawing.

Practice of this technique requires a basic understanding of anatomy, homeopathics, dousing, a clear mind, and study with a trained Radionics practitioner.

I had two separate Radionics broadcasts performed on me during a 12-month period. The first treatment was for a variety of ailments. I followed the prescribed regimen which included Radionics broadcasts to me in Austin from Albuquerque and taking homeopathic supplements. I was sent periodic updates on how my condition was progressing. The first time I had Radionics performed I could not definitively confirm that it was working. My intuition told me that there were benefits being received, but no real tangible evidence. I just had to take Terry's word for it.

The second time I had a Radionics treatment I received proof positive that it had worked. I volunteer at a shelter for at risk children every Sunday. One week there was a group of children who had ring worm, a common fungus that shows up on your skin as a ring shaped rash. I came into contact with the ring worms while playing with the children, but did not think I had gotten it since I regularly wash my hands when at the shelter.

I visited Terry a few days after being exposed. She performed a Radethesia evaluation and immediatcly detected that I had ring worm. She set up a Radionics broadcast for me and prescribed an herbal anti-fungal remedy to treat the ring worm. There was no way Terry could have known about them, since there was no visual indication.

A few days after my visit, I noticed ring-shaped rashes, indicative of ring worm, on my stomach that itched. I went to a naturopath in Austin for a physical. Using the Asyra bio energetic diagnostic equipment, it was immediately confirmed that I had ring worm, which, was winding down as a result of the herbs and the broadcasts. The naturopath concurred that the rashes on my stomach were from the ring worm. The condition was gone just a few days later. This was my proof that Radethesia and Radionics work.

I will let Terry Kast tell you more about Radionics in her own words, since I have just scratched the surface. I think this is really cool stuff that is worth of sharing with you.

Energy Healing Through Radionics[1] – Terry Kast

What if you could send a sample of your blood from a mere finger prick to a health practitioner to learn some amazing information about your health issues? What if the practitioner could actually use that sample of blood to send corrective, healing energy to you to help you alleviate your problem? And what if you could learn to do it all for yourself, eliminating the guess work and cutting through all the hype and contradictory advice that is out there? Think this is impossible? Think again. People are already doing it. The type of work is called Radionics. Here is how it works:

An electromagnetic field pervades every cell throughout your body. This field contains variations in frequency. Valerie Hunt, PhD, retired physiology professor from U.C.L.A. has studied this field and established these frequencies. She has concluded that a strong, healthy field is key to one's health and energy. She says that your energetic field not only is acted upon by the environment (and its toxins), but that your field interacts with the environment. Energy healing teaches us that because of this interaction with the environment, a strong energetic field which is well-represented at all

---

1   Kast, Terry, *Parcells Method of Healing*, P.O. Box 50010, Albuquerque, NM 87181

levels of frequency can help to protect you from toxins, increasing your resistance to disease and toxicity, itself. It appears that a strong energetic field is a vital part of the body's immune system.

The body's energy field has been photographed by many through Kirlian photography. Dr. Hunt has tested this field in the laboratory to verify its existence and learn more about its relationship to sickness and health. She has concluded that in order to be healthy, one must cultivate and maintain a strong, healthy energetic field that is well represented in frequency. More details of her work are available through her website and by purchasing her video, *Understanding Energy Fields*.

How does one get a healthy field? Certainly everything you do to help your body can help this process. Nutrition, exercise, healthy living habits, and positive thinking are basic. Natural healing methods such as chiropractic, herbal medicine, homeopathy, and acupuncture are basic to healthy living and help to support energy flow throughout your body. I think all natural therapies can help enhance the energy field. But one of the most dependable and dramatic ways to get a strong, balanced energy field is through Radionics. In fact, it is one of the most amazing ways to heal.

What is Radionics?

Radionics is the transmission of energy through an electromagnetic field to effect a beneficial, balancing change in the body's electromagnetic field. Since we have this energy field that pervades every cell in the body and thus, runs throughout the entire body, it is only logical that by affecting this field appropriately-with the right healing agents – that one can affect the tissues of the body itself. This is, in effect, what Radionics accomplishes.

Many of us have experienced different forms of energy healing that is accomplished by the practitioner's "hands on" approach, such as Therapeutic Touch or Reiki. In Radionics, no one touches the person or animal being worked on. In fact, in most cases, when the healing and energy balancing is being performed, the person or animal is not even present! This is because, in Radionics, the energetic balancing that transpires is conducted through an electromagnetic field and goes to the person or animal through a blood, or saliva sample from that being. The blood and saliva contain DNA, as we know. Radionics demonstrates that the blood and saliva contain the body's energetic imprint that is unique to that individual. This energetic imprint becomes the contact point as the energetic corrections travel through the earth's magnetic field to make contact in the person's electromagnetic field. This contact is instant because, there is no distance in space and time in this context of physics. Some of my students who are engineers have said that this is the closest demonstration of quantum physics that they have ever encountered. You can learn more about this concept by reading a book entitled, *Science and Human Transformation*, by William Tiller, PhD, where he explains the physics behind this incredible occurrence.

The idea of energy traveling to contact someone, regardless of distance sounds impossible, yet we think nothing of wireless transmission in radio, cell phone or computer technology-because it is common place and we accept it. The technology for this form of healing has been around since the early 1900's and has been kept underground because it was suppressed and its practitioners persecuted by the American Medical Association and the Food and Drug Administration. The reasons for the suppression and persecution by these establishments have been, of course, economic. Today, more and more people are discovering healing benefits from Radionics and discovering that there is more potential for health and healing than we ever thought possible.

I came into this form of healing, when my husband, a chiropractor, was diagnosed with an incurable disease. A friend of mine was taking her second course from Dr. Hazel Parcells, a naturopath and chiropractor, who had developed her own method of Radionics. Dr. Parcells had developed a method of targeting specific areas of the body for detoxification and energetic support. Dr. Parcells method excels on accuracy and her use of magnetic fields is highly effective-especially in detoxification of the body, because she developed the capability of working on the denser electromagnetic field that is closest to the body.

I later learned that other methods of Radionics work more on the more subtle fields, so I was fortunate that my first encounter with Radionics has been one of the best.

My friend used this process called "broadcasting" to help my husband everyday during the week of their Radionics class. She had my husband's blood sample at Dr. Parcell's office downtown, while my husband was at home several miles away. Broadcasting is done routinely without the person being present! During that time, my husband began to make some progress. I really thought my friend had "lost it" because these ideas were so foreign to me, but I could not deny what I saw happening to him. His color and energy had improved and he was able to participate in more activities around the home. My friend continued "broadcasting" to him after the Radionics class was over. She would call me with instructions for nutritional supplements or homeopathics or detoxification baths. I followed her instructions.

Within a few weeks of continued work-especially the "broadcasting," his blood tests began to change. Within 6 weeks, he was back working half days in his chiropractic office. My friend had convinced me to start taking classes from Dr. Parcells. I was soon able to do the "broadcasting" for my husband, and within a month, he was able to work full-time. That was in 1978 and he has NEVER had a recurrence of this potentially terminal disease.

I continued to study with Dr. Parcells throughout the 1980s and for several months in 1990–91, had the pleasure of working with her full-time, where I could continue to learn what she was not ready to bring into class. She was working on a way to incorporate other radionics units with the unit that she had developed to be able to reach more levels of frequencies. I have continued this effort with radionics and today we can reach a far wider range of frequencies, which give us far greater healing capability.

This method of healing has become a way of life for us and changed our perception of health and illness. Our reality is truly different. We do not have most of the limitations that most people experience regarding health. Dr. Parcells taught that a disease is simply the name of a condition that describes what your body is doing about what you are doing or have been exposed to. She used a process called Radiesthesia, a form of energetic testing done with a stainless steel pendulum in a magnetic field, to determine energetic blockages, which would usually turn out to be contributing factors, causing the problem. The causes are usually toxins that have layered deeply into the body's tissues and organ structures that compromise normal function of the areas involved. Until my husband became ill, I had no idea how many horrific toxins we are exposed to everyday. Not all of us can throw these toxins off. Some people, like my husband, absorb them and become hopelessly ill.

When students would tell Dr. Parcells that they had an illness, she would teach us how to perform our energetic testing to determine causation. Then, through broadcasting to these students—sending the appropriate energy to them—through an electro-magnetic field— we would observe the improvements. The method of Radionics that Dr.Parcells had developed would literally neutralize the toxins in targeted areas of the body. These toxins are apparently dissolved at the molecular level and do not end up in your blood stream having to be "processed" by your liver, kidneys or intestinal tract.

The advantage of that is that there is no further risk of those toxins being reabsorbed by the body in those areas-as is frequently the case when taking herbal detoxification formulas or undergoing chelation therapies. You don't feel tired as you often would when these toxins are having to travel through your system and be processed through the pathways of elimination. It is so wonderful to take care of detoxification at this energetic, molecular level. When the toxins are neutralized in this way, the molecular composition of the toxins are apparently broken up and the physical substance is changed into a substance that the body is able to process. Broadcasting has been going on since the early or mid 1900s. and its effects have been entirely beneficial. Dr. Parcells had heard of no negative reports of reactions of any kind in all of the years that she was developing her part of this work. In all of the years that I have been involved since 1978, I have only observed beneficial, positive changes. We are thankful to my friend and Dr. Parcells for their diligence in bringing this form of healing to us. It has been an incredible experience that has changed our lives and has helped us to help others.

Today, if I don't like the way I feel, I test myself through this evaluation system, which I have advanced and clarified for my students. I use a stainless steel pendulum in an electromagnetic field to determine what is going on and what I need to do to turn things around. It is a phenomenal method of "self help"! My students and I no longer have to depend on others. We can determine the best supplements, herbs, homeopathic and other health agents for ourselves and our loved ones. We can determine what our bodies need to restore balance and we can broadcast ourselves or our loved ones to help us feel better fast! The broadcasts neutralize and eliminate toxins, eliminating pain and fatigue in the process! The broadcasting is truly miraculous. My students have done incredible things. They have saved their loved ones from surgeries, saved limbs from amputation, saved teeth from extraction or root canals, and restored health and energy when all hope was lost. They have recovered from chronic fatigue and fibromyalgia and effected healthy changes in their mental and emotional health, as well.

In 1994, Dr. Parcells moved out of Albuquerque to a mountain village north of Santa Fe, NM. She was 104. She was still talking to groups who would visit her, but doing very little broadcasting herself. In 1996, Dr. Parcells died at the age of 106. A book entitled, Live Better Longer, was published about her and some of her ideas about health. It is a valuable resource, but does not delve very much into the energetic aspects of disease. That is where I come in. My students and I have been preserving the work of this great practitioner and researcher. We help to empower people in these methods to do their own healing with our teaching and guidance.

Here are some of our real life stories:[1]

'Several years ago, my father had a heart attack and stroke. He was in ICU on a respirator and on kidney dialysis. After he had been there about a week, I got a blood sample and began working with Terry to send him energy to his heart and lungs. He was off the respirator the day after beginning the process. We then focused on sending energy to the kidneys. He was off dialysis the following day. This work helped ease his suffering and helped to get him out of ICU. I have also had other dramatic experiences regarding Terry's methods. Her work helped my son, when he had a severe case of pneumonia. He was able to get well without having to go through a procedure for draining the fluid off of his lungs, which had been a real possibility during his illness.

We have also helped an elderly family member avoid an amputation of a leg, which had been scheduled for amputation. Terry's energetic work was done within days of the scheduled surgery. I have used this work many times for my own healing.

---

1   Kast, Terry, *Parcells Method of Healing*, P.O. Box 50010, Albuquerque, NM 87181

147   Rich Remedies

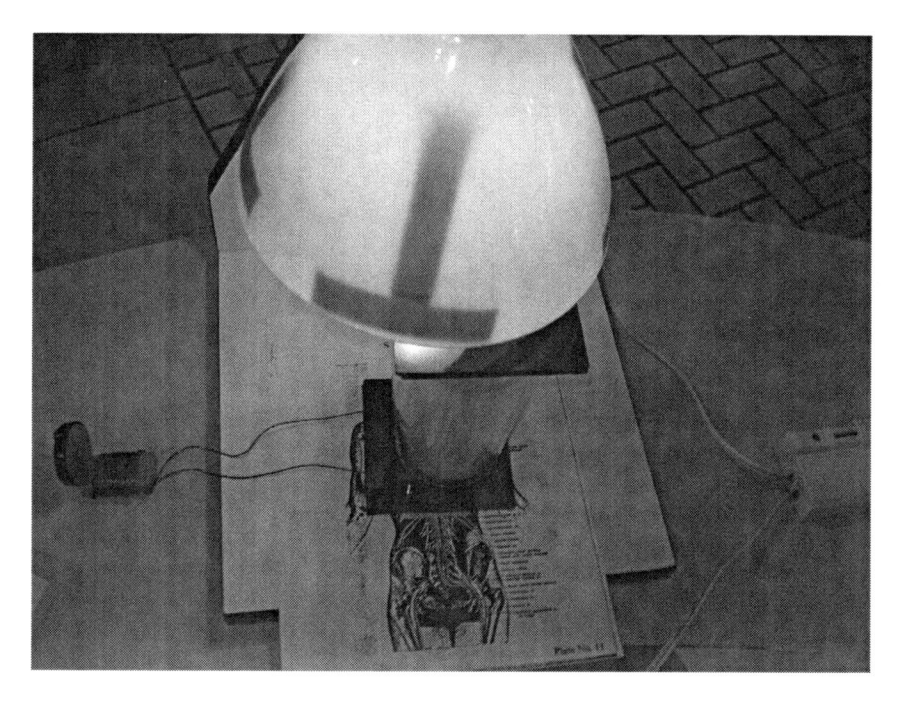

This is the configuration for the Radionics broadcast to treat my ring worm and several other issues, which was done while in Albuquerque, New Mexico. It's amazing.

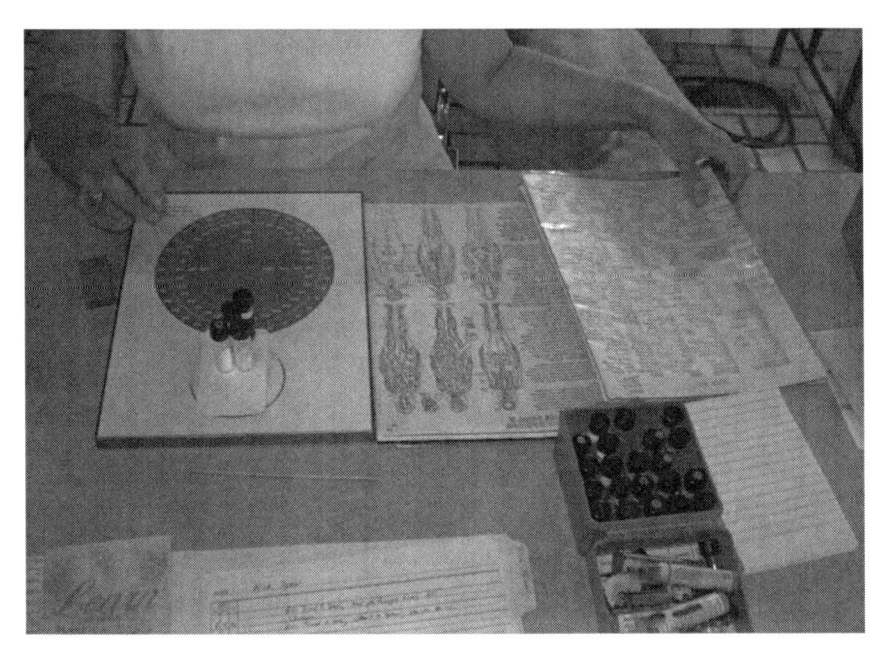

This is the Radiesthesia energetic testing tablet, anatomical illustrations, and homeopathics. As discussed in my experience, ring worm was detected in my body and then appeared on my skin several days later. I had my doubts about this technique until this condition was detected and then successfully treated using Radionics. I was and am still amazed by this experience.

Bill W., D.D.S., N.M.D., Albuquerque, NM

"I first came to Terry's class in Albuquerque in 1997. I had been suffering from chronic fatigue syndrome and had basically been sick in one way or another most of my life. I have always used alternative therapies, hoping to find some answers for my chronic health problems. I began working with Terry during that class and kept up the work. I was amazed. I made more progress in 3 months than I had in 30 years! This work has helped me with fatigue, "brain fog," digestive problems and parasites, immune situations and has brought me out of some serious infec¬tions. Terry's work has helped me keep my health so that I can travel and do what I have to do. I have continued with this work and use it almost every day."

Ellen G., Tucson AZ

"I am a close friend of Terry's and have had the good fortune to have benefited from her work many times. A couple of years ago, I was airlifted from my local hospital to a hospital in Albuquerque, NM. CT scans had revealed a massive abdominal infection and stones in the pancreas. I was put on IV's for infection and told that they would do surgery as soon as the infection was under control. I called my friend and she did broadcasts to me for the infection and for the stones. A few days later, they did a pre-surgical MRI to determine the state of the infection and the stones. They were very surprised to see that not only was all of the infection gone, but the stones were gone, too! I asked them if they could tell me what happened and they said they did not know. They were very shocked and could not explain how I had gotten well so fast! I was dismissed without surgery. Of course, I did not tell them what my friend was doing- they would not have believed it anyway. But I know what happened. I could feel it while the broadcasts were working. Because of this work, I did not have to have surgery!"

Larissa T., Gallup, NM

"When I first called Terry Kast and became her student, I had been suffering from chronic fatigue syndrome for many years. My memory was poor, my energy low, and my ability to focus was difficult. I looked 10 years older than I was. As I became involved in this method of healing, Terry helped me recover from heavy metal poisoning and helped me detoxify-both through supplements and from energetic healing done through radionics, which we learned how to do for ourselves in class. I have experienced much healing through this method over the years, because I have come to understand that detoxification is an on-going process. This work has helped me to recover from chronic fatigue, so that I could do my life's work. It has given me the energy to write my book, to create, to travel, to give talks, and to start another book! It has also helped me test foods and supplements I might need to take."

"Having experienced the "broadcasting," of radionics, the connection between the blood sample and receptor is very real to me. I describe it to others as a cell phone calling all over the USA or the world...no one else's phone rings when dialed. The energy needed reaches the person represented by the blood sample. I have experienced so much healing support from this method and over so many years, that I am convinced that this method is a viable tool for health and healing. It has helped me and several members of my family, immensely."

Nancy B., Santa Fe, New Mexico

So these are some real world examples of how radionics and radthesia work in healing. It's just nature at work. Everything has an electromagnetic frequency. All Radionics does is treat disease with a frequency that neutralizes it and, in many cases, this is being accomplished over long distances.

Edgar Cayce, whose work is covered in the next chapter, successfully practiced long distance healing for over 30 years and has over 14,000 written case studies to prove it. Radionics is just another technique to accomplish healing in a very unique and effective way. Believe it or not!

Chapter 15
Effective Microorganisms™
The Power of Magnetic Wave Resonance

A healing solution that is proven and defies all common sense and scientific logic.

I had completed the manuscript for Rich Remedies Volume 1, after delaying its completion to add the short story of Phosphatidylcholine Choline in Chapter 4., Vitamins and Nutrition. This project had already drifted six months past my original completion date ,so I had committed to myself that any additional healing discoveries would have to wait for the sequel to this book, *Rich Remedies Volume 2*. But instead, I found Effective Microorganisms™ (EM™) and decided that the printing presses had to stop, yet again, to include a short description of this powerful, energetic healing solution.

My discovery of EM™ was another "accident". I was looking for a few quotes from Masaru Emoto in his book, The Secret Life of Water, when I stumbled upon references to "Hado" and "Hado Medicine".1 As I read further I realized that he was referring to the basic premise of this book that everything has a vibration, frequency, and resonance. His term for using energy is "Hado". This concept has a different name everywhere in the world, but refers to the same thing, which is the conscious use of life energy. This is yet another data point in my growing collection of data points that supports the discoveries that I made in natural healing and how the energy of things plays into all of them.

EM™ is part of Dr. Emoto's set of Hado examples in The Secret Life of Water. He discusses at length the incredible results that were being seen around the world as part of Dr. Teru Higa's work in using EM™ in environmental cleanup, agriculture, construction, and other applications. Since I'm on a crusade to find cool healing things, I immediately did a web search on Dr. Higa and EM™ to learn more. What I discovered amazed me and motivated me to get involved in using EM™ and distributing the products.

"EM Technology™ is the use of antioxidants, enzymes, and other bio-available compounds derived from fermentation of a specific culture of microorganisms to exert beneficial effects on the surrounding environment. The technology was developed by Dr. Teruo Higa, a professor of horticulture at the University of the Ryukyus in Okinawa, Japan. EM Technology™ is used in making several patented products ranging from various water treatment devices to jewelry, textiles, plastics, and building materials."[2]

"EM•1® Microbial Inoculant is a liquid containing many co-existing microorganisms. The major groups of microorganisms in EM•1® Microbial Inoculant are lactic acid bacteria, yeast, and phototropic bacteria. EM™ was first developed in 1982 as an alternative to synthetic chemicals in the field of agriculture. Through extensive research and experiments over time, EM™ became recognized as effective in various fields, including environmental remediation, recycling organic wastes, reducing odor in livestock operations, treating wastewater, and many more."[3]

A significant body of research recorded at the EM Research Organization in Japan supports all of the incredible applications and use cases that are attributed to EM Technology™. Time does not permit me to delve deeply into them, here as this will be included in-depth in *Rich Remedies Volume 2*, where I will have had at least one year of personal experience and research to validate what I already intuitively believe to be true about EM Technology™.

[1] Emoto, Masaru. *The Secret Life of Water.* Hillsboro, Ore.: Beyond Words Publishing, Inc., 2003. Page 50.

[2] EM America, Alto, Texas

[3] EM Research Organization, Inc emrojapan.com

My understanding of EM™ is as follows—the microbes in EM•1® Microbial Inoculant are "probiotics for the Earth". Like the beneficial probiotics that I take to keep "bad" bacteria in check in my digestive system, the EM•1® Microbial Inoculant does the same thing, only on a much broader scale. In Dr. Higa's book, Our Future Reborn, he explains how we have forces of syntropy (positive energy, life-giving) effects and entropy (negative energy, destructive) effects on nature and our world. In the invisible world of microorganisms, Dr. Higa observed that 10% are "good", beneficial to life and 10% are "bad", destructive to life, while the other 80% are "uncommitted". Like spectators in the human race, the "uncommitted" are watching the action from the sidelines and will jump in on the side of the winning team once they can determine who has the momentum and the will to win.[4]

So to take my metaphor further, EM™ is the champ in every encounter. It has a "knock out punch" that the "bad bacteria" can't handle. It has what Dr. Higa calls magnetic wave resonance. This is an incredible syntropic healing energy. I call it "Ki on steroids".
It defies all common sense and scientific logic. This is one of the reasons I like EM Technology™, because like many of the things I embrace, there is no "science" to completely explain it. Just boatloads of research and documented evidence on its successful application in solving many of the world's pressing problems.

EM™ will confound right brain thinkers, scientists, and engineers because it's efficacy and application defies our collective experience. It delights left brain thinkers like me. It sounds too good to be true. You can't see magnetic wave resonance, just the results that it delivers. It confounds all the modern thinking and scientific logic. I love it! The people who think what I have written in this book is a bunch of "hooey" will really dislike EM™, because they can't comprehend it, will want to dismiss it, and then will have to accept it in the face of a large library of evidence that it really works. The

---

4   Higa, Teruo, PhD.Our Future Reborn. Tokyo, Japan:Sunmark Publishing. 2006.

proof is in real, tangible, results.

"EM™ absorbs energy. It appears to absorb free form energy from an external source. This mechanism is similar to when plants use carbon dioxide and solar energy to synthesize substances, resulting in powerful energy.[5] In the case of EM™, this mechanism is thought to involve a strong antioxidizing function simultaneously combined with the wave effect that absorbs energy from an unidentified source. There are many types of wave motion, but EM™ wave motion is believed to have ultra high frequency, ultra low energy magnetic wave resonance qualities that defy common sense. Although further study is required, EM™'s effects on dioxin and radiation, natural healing powers and energy-conservation properties cannot be explained without this peculiar **magnetic wave resonance**."

So this citation makes everything crystal clear to you, doesn't it?

Success stories abound in Dr. Higa's wonderful book, *Our Future Reborn*. It is required reading. One of the most incredible stories was the restoration of the Seto Inland Sea with EM.[6] This massive cleanup project started with the formation of a taskforce to educate the public and to gain acceptance and usage of EM™-based products for sewage disposal, dioxin pollution remediation, soil remediation, and direct infusions of EM™ into estuaries and the Seto Inland Sea which was extremely polluted. The fish, shellfish, and seaweed populations were miniscule due to residential, agricultural, and industrial pollution. EM™ was introduced into all of these sectors for the treatment of wastes. They also set up a massive fermentation system to produce EM•1® Microbial Inoculant in quantities to support wide use and to dump directly into the polluted sea.

In just five years the nearly lifeless Seto Inland Sea was teaming with schools of fish. The shellfish populations were at pre-industrial

---

5   Higa, Teruo, PhD. *Our Future Reborn*. Tokyo, Japan: Sunmark Publishing. 2006. Pages 162–162.

6   Higa, Teruo, PhD. *Our Future Reborn*. Tokyo, Japan: Sunmark Publishing. 2006. Pages 38–44.

pollution levels. Octopus returned, and the seaweed beds were producing clean, fresh, edible product once again. I have never heard of this large-scale pollution remediation success before. I find it almost unbelievable, but it is all documented.

Another huge success story was the restoration of North Korean agriculture that had been destroyed by years of chemical farming and soil depletion. The North Korean situation created famine and human suffering on a massive scale that was well-publicized in newspapers around the globe. This crisis and human suffering were eventually averted through the use of EM Technology™ in farming across the country. This is a little known fact. I do not support the politics of the North Korean government, but I do condone assisting innocent, starving people. EM™ played a major role in ending the famine and suffering. There are many more stories like this.

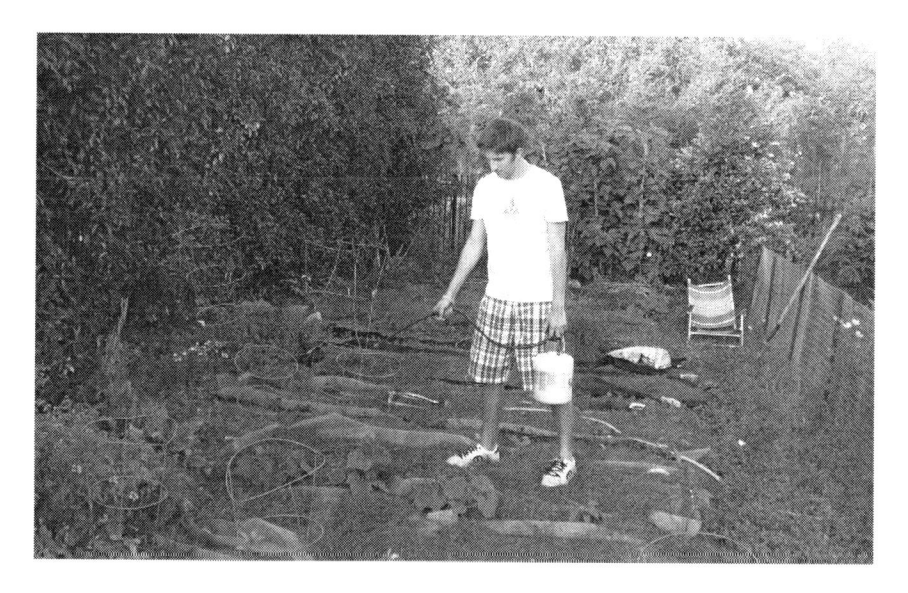

This photo shows EM•1® Microbial Inoculants being sprayed on my organic garden to improve soil microorganism activity. This process increases crop yield and soil fertility.

EM™ has broad applications as mentioned before and are identified by their brand names:

EM•1® Microbial Inoculants: Applications in agriculture, wastewater treatment, composting, odor control, bioremediation, phytoremediation, construction, and aquaculture.

PRO EM•1® Daily Probotic Cleanse: Nutritional probiotics for digestive health

EM•X® Rice Bran Extract: A nutritional health drink for improved health with high magnetic wave resonance.

EM•X® Ceramics: Energy absorbing and radiating materials EM Technology™ — The application of EM™ too many secondary uses in technology and healthcare.

My Experience

Having just discovered EM™, my experience is limited to the personal use of EM•1® Microbial Inoculant for my organic garden, PRO EM•1® Daily Probiotic Cleanse for daily nutritional use, EM•X® Rice Bran Extract for daily nutritional supplementation, and EM•X® Ceramics for light jewelry. I was so impressed by the potential of EM™ that I am offering it through my website. I recommend that you check out my website located in the Resources section at the end of this book. *Rich Remedies Volume 2* will have a more detailed chapter on my personal experiences with EM™. I expect the results to be very positive. Stay tuned.

SECTION 3
TWO HEALING LEGENDS
HAZEL PARCELLS & EDGAR CAYCE

Chapter 16
Dr. Hazel Parcells, PhD

Hazel Parcells, who lived to be 107 years old, cured herself, at the age of 42, of "terminal" tuberculosis and then dedicated herself to the natural healing arts for the next 65 years. She was a pioneer in natural healing, a lady way ahead of her time.

She bucked the system when it came to most common allopathic medicine treatment regimens, favoring natural remedies. Periodically she came under attack from conventional medicine bureaucrats, who felt threatened by her gentle, natural, and effective healing techniques. She was in many cases, like Edgar Cayce - the healing solution of last resort for very ill people. A lot of her patients had been written off by conventional physicians and went to Dr. Parcells just before preparing their Last Will and Testaments. More often than not, she succeeded in providing her patients with relief. The human body has a tremendous capability to heal itself if given the right nutrients and energetic stimulation, as Parcells consistently demonstrated in her practice.

Like many of the good folks that I have met in the natural healing arts, she was said to be quirky and a bit eccentric based on first-hand accounts from people who studied under her. Being a good healer does not require a "conventional appearance or lifestyle" as I have found out. They just have to be good at what they do, have compassion for their patients, and be committed to continuing education so they can keep up with new technologies and techniques. Dr. Parcells' life focus was on the good work of healing people, not documenting, publishing, and disseminating her great discoveries to the world at large. Hence, her incredible work is generally unknown.

She was an outside-of-the-box, inventive thinker who discovered healing tips and methods that I had never considered or heard mentioned by today's well-known nutritional experts. She spent years studying nature and extracting healing solutions from decades of observation and clinical experimentation.

The most interesting things that she brought to my awareness were the prevalence and dangers of parasites, heavy metals, and radiation in our daily environment. The healing possibilities of radionics (covered in Chapter 14), full spectrum light (Chapter 12), cleansing (Chapter 6), and therapeutic color (Chapter 12) are other techniques that I have latched on to and incorporated into my own healing bag of tricks. I do these for fun, not out of fear or some hypochondria.

My discovery of Hazel Parcells' work was accidental (even though I believe there really are no accidents). I found a macrobiotic news journal in a health food store that discussed the Parcells' food cleanse for getting chemicals out of food and killing bacteria. This is used all over the world in developing countries by relief workers concerned about getting sick from local water and food. A few days after seeing this article, I saw a reference to Parcells in Jacob Lieberman's book *Light Medicine of the Future* where he referenced her use of light and color as part of healing. So in my tradition of making a line from two dots of information, I started researching Hazel Parcells. This lead me to *Live Better Longer* by Joseph Dispenza, a gem of a book on taking charge of your own healing, that documents many of Dr. Parcells' healing discoveries.

Hazel Parcells used what I call "Cosmic Folk Medicine;" a mixture of natural folk medicine, intuition, metaphysics, clinical laboratory trials, and common sense. Through these combined activities she found the key to the healing secrets of nature.

Once I got the book, *Live Better Longer: The Parcells Center 7-Step Plan for Health and Longevity*, I called the Parcells Center in Santa Fe, NM, and found out that it had shuttered its doors. Upon further research I found that the remnants of the Parcells Center had relocated to Albuquerque, New Mexico and was operated by Terry Kast, who had been a student of Dr. Parcells.

Terry is a terrific person, full of energy and spirit and just as dedicated to the healing arts as Dr. Parcells. When we first spoke, I was just interested in ordering colored glass and a prism to check out some of Dr. Parcells's recommendations on using these energies for healing. Our discussion shifted gears quickly when she told me about using dousing for diagnosing illness and then broadcast a remedy. These natural healing techniques are called radiesthesia (diagnosis) and radionics (broadcasting homeopathics). To me this stuff is real "magic," although in reality it is not magic, just nature at work. We should never be surprised by nature's potential. In my brief encounter with the Native American healing art of Drum Washing I found the same "magic" energy at work. It is available to all of us who are capable and willing to tap into the Earth's energy fields and Universal Intelligence.

This stuff has been around for centuries. We in the West have been de-sensitized to this energy by all of our modern distractions, conveniences, and institutional dis-information. Deeply spiritual people, or "conscious" people like Native American Shamans, tap into these energies all of the time.

My Experience

Parcells Oxygen Soak[1]

Registered with the Smithsonian Institution under Simplified Kitchen Chemistry I'm told that United Nations relief workers around the world use this.

After the multiple outbreaks of salmonella poisoning, green

---

1 Dispenza, Joseph. *Live Better Longer: The Parcells Center 7-Step Plan for Health and Longevity.* Lincoln, Nebr: iUniverse.com, Inc. 2000 Pages 43–44.

onion contamination, contaminated processed meat recalls, and all the pesticides used in industrial agriculture, this is probably a good measure to take while cleaning your food here in the US.

1 Teaspoon of Clorox bleach to 1 gallon of water

Description	Soaking time
Leafy Vegetables	5–10 mins.
Root vegetables	10–15 mins.
Fruits: Thin-skinned fruits, such as berries	5 mins.
Medium skinned fruits, such as peaches, apricots and plums	10 mins.
Thick-skinned fruits, such as apples	10–15 mins.
Citrus fruits and bananas	15 mins.
Eggs	20–30 mins.
Meat/Poultry	15–20 mins.

Rinse in clean water for 10 to 15 minutes.

The Parcels soak is said to oxygenate, food, giving it a fresher taste and longer refrigerator shelf life. (I've noticed the refrigerator shelf life has increased for some produce, but no guarantees here. What I am confident of is that the food I am eating is really clean.)

Food contamination in the US is a huge issue, causing much sickness. You would think that, with the FDA and other watchdog groups working on consumer safety, factory food would be safe. However, with big business involved and profits at stake, your family's health becomes a secondary concern. So take it upon yourself to protect your family from agricultural chemicals and contaminated food by using this simple, but effective, cleaning recipe. It's probably better than what most of us are doing now.

The Parcells soak is also a good way for people with no access to organically grown food to purify the industrially grown produce that they eat. Organic produce is expensive, and in some areas virtually impossible to buy at the local supermarket. The soak can improve the quality and cleanliness of just about any produce.

My Experience

I do this with all fruits and vegetables (when time permits), especially the ones that have caused salmonella scares like green onions and spinach. After you soak some fruits and vegetables you will notice a scum or coating on the top of the used Clorox water. These are chemicals, wax, and pesticides that you and your children would have otherwise eaten. These chemicals accumulate in the body eventually making you sick or compromising your immune system. It's a good precaution to remove as many of these chemicals as possible from your foods before eating them and then, periodically, doing an internal cleansing to get rid of the ones that you do consume. You can never avoid environmental toxins, but this is a way to reduce your consumption.

The soak can be time consuming, so I buy my vegetables for the week and do this just one time. If my veggies are coming from a trusted, local organic farm, I generally will not soak them. However, produce from big supermarket chains always gets soaked, especially spinach and green onions. Any time vegetables are grown in close proximity to grazing lands or are fertilized with animal waste, you are at risk for salmonella poisoning. Since you, as the consumer, have no way of knowing this, precautions are sometimes prudent in the preparation of vegetables.

Therapeutic Bathing[2]

This has nothing to do with bath houses, so please don't get alarmed. No public bathing or mixing with naked people required!

Parcell's says this helps dissipate the energy draining effects of radiation.

I travel on airplanes a lot and am exposed to radiation from the high altitude flying and the X-ray equipment at airports. After a particularly grueling multi-city trip, where I have been constantly zapped with radiation, I soak in a hot tub of water mixed with 1 pound of baking soda and 1 pound of sea salt, for 45 minutes to an hour. I think it works because I feel invigorated after one of these detox baths.

The Use of Color Therapy[3]

I have no clue if color water or rainbow water actually works. What I can tell you is that you do have color and light coursing through every molecule of your body so, color supplementation makes sense to me, though I can't prove that there is anything here. I just do it. The laughs (at my expense) from my children that I get preparing color water alone are worth the effort. There's healing in their laughter. You see, I don't take anything too seriously.

Here's how you get some laughs and some colored water:

Take a glass of distilled or filtered tap water and place a small pane of colored cathedral glass or colored plastic photo gels over the top of the glass for 30 minutes. Place the glass in full sunlight or under a full spectrum light. To get rainbow water repeat the same step with a prism. Drink water and have a good laugh. If nothing else, it's good for a laugh which is very important.

---

2   Dispenza, Joseph. *Live Better Longer: The Parcells Center 7-Step Plan for Health and Longevity.* Lincoln, Nebr: iUniverse.com, Inc. 2000 Pages 29–34.

3   Dispenza, Joseph. *Live Better Longer: The Parcells Center 7-Step Plan for Health and Longevity.* Lincoln, Nebr: iUniverse.com, Inc. 2000. Pages 128–135.

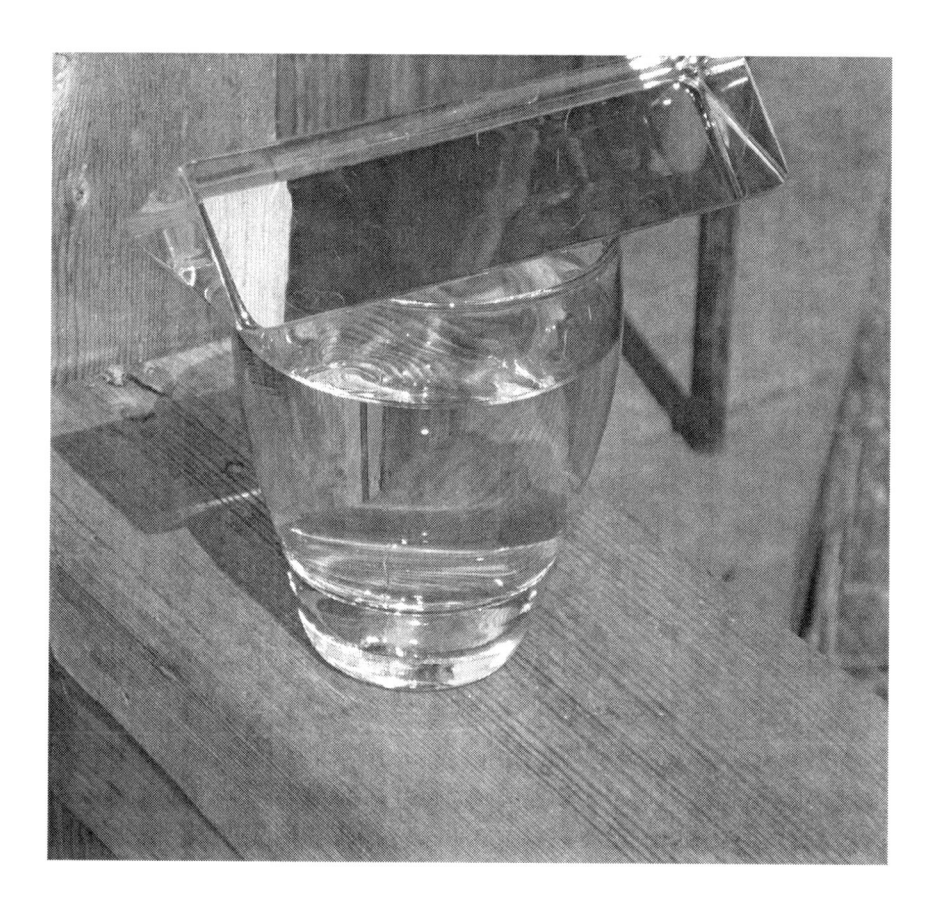

Using Full Spectrum Light[4]

Dr. Parcells was a leader in the use of full spectrum light and color as a holistic approach to healing. She was conscious of every dimension of how to treat the human energy field. Full spectrum light is close to the sun's light and therefore promotes the growth and nourishment of living things. It is the best way to light a room for mood enhancement, production of vitamin D, learning, and growing live plants.

---

4   Dispenza, Joseph. *Live Better Longer: The Parcells Center 7-Step Plan for Health and Longevity.* Lincoln, Nebr: iUniverse.com, Inc. 2000. Pages 133–134.

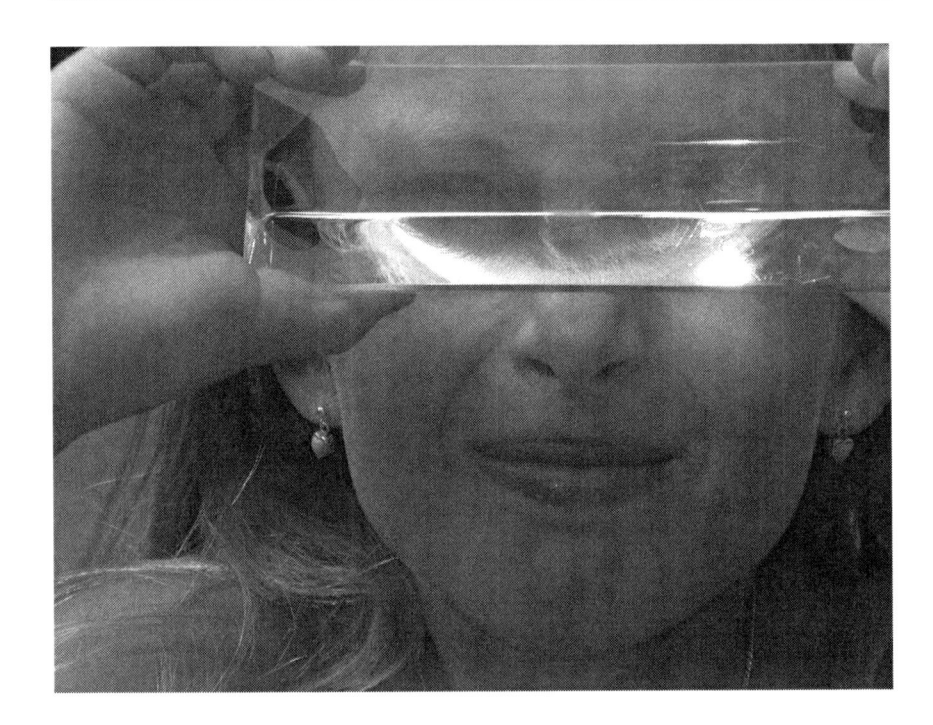

This photo shows full spectrum light color being taken directly into the eyes through a glass prism. Dr. Parcells said that if there was only one healing tool she could keep, it would be color. She was known to carry a glass prism with her and when travelling would take "color breaks" to re-energize her body. A more complete discussion can be found in Chapter 14.

Electromagnetic Fields (EMFs)

There is a lot in the news these days about the dangers of long-term exposure to EMFs (gretar than 2.0 milligaus) generated by cell phones, televisions, wireless computer networks, microwave towers, X-ray machines, CAT Scans, high tension electric power lines, radar, and other invisible energy pollutants. Parcells was well aware of the disruptive effects that EMFs have on the human energy field and those of other animals For most of us it's out-of-sight, out-of-mind.

She recommended avoiding or reducing exposure to EMF sources, taking therapeutic baths, internal cleansing, and radionics to help reduce the effects of EMF"s. Like other environmental pollutants, you can't avoid EMFs in a modern, industrialized society, but you can cut your exposure and detoxify.

The aspect of Parcell's work that was particularly enlightening and alarming to me is the prevalence of radioactive fallout from atomic bomb testing that still exists in our environment. Since the first atomic bombs were tested, then used on the Japanese at Hiroshima during World War II, radioactive particles have been released into the Earth's atmosphere and blown by the four winds across the earth to every continent.

Pro-nuclear pundits will tell you that the trace amounts of radioactive dust that are in the environment from atomic bomb detonation are less harmful than the natural radiation you get from sunlight or a flight on an airplane. After all the BS that I have been fed by the "authorities" on how EMFs are harmless, I choose to believe that they are lying and that people like Hazel Parcells and Terry Kast are telling me the truth. The experts have been BSing all of us for years on many fronts, but particularly on military matters. I do think that "ignorance is bliss" in some areas, otherwise we'd all be basket cases worrying constantly about what we are exposed to on a daily basis.

Unfortunately, everything that is done in every corner of this world does affect us, whether we want to acknowledge it or not. I don't suggest people freak out, just be aware that it's happening and know the precautions you can take to reduce the damage to you and your family.

These invisible, harmful frequencies weren't around in the good old days, so some of the increases in terminal diseases may be due to all the different EMFs, including radiation, that modern society is exposed to. I don't know; it's just a guess on my part. There are credible scientists who will tell you all of this concern about EMFs is a complete crock. You can believe them if you choose. I choose not to.

An interesting story related to the presence of radiation in our environment appeared in an issue of the *Wall Street Journal*. It was about how a wealthy wine collector who was sold a Napoleonic-era (or so it was advertised) bottle of French wine for $100,000. He had a sample of the wine tested at a laboratory for authenticity. They lab tested it for the presence of radiation and found some traces, thus determining that the bottle was bogus.

It turns out that all wines grown after 1945 (the year that the atomic bomb was dropped) will show minute traces of radiation. This is very revealing. What does that tell you? "It's a small world after all." This stuff is everywhere. Just hope that a big cloud doesn't fall into your back yard!

What alarmed me was the pocket of radiation detected by Terry Kast in the left chamber of my heart. I had a radionics treatment to remove it, but was shocked to learn that this silent killer was just sitting there, slowly poisoning me. Terry told me that every time a country sets off an atomic explosion, the effects are felt (literally) around the world, resulting in some cases, in personal contamination.

To protect myself in some small measure from environmental radiation, I take therapeutic baths, eat kelp, which contains natural iodine (good for radiation poisoning), and get radionics. The risks of radiation poisoning are probably not that great unless you get a good dose. The problem is that radiation, like all EMFs, is invisible, so you don't know you've been zapped until you get really sick, and then, sometimes, it's too late.

I probably sound like an alarmist here, and in actual fact I don't dwell on radiation, I just like being conscious that it is around, that we're all being exposed to it. This information enables me to take some very minor and convenient precautions to reduce radiation's effect on me.

In closing, Hazel Parcels is a healing legend who deserves more recognition and credit than she has received by the mass media. More importantly, her recommendations for using nature to heal ourselves should be incorporated into our daily lives for optimum health.

"All life on our planet depends for nourishment on light from the sun; a critical balance of visible color and invisible ultraviolet wavelengths ... the essence of life in energy is color."

— Dr. Hazel Parcells

Chapter 17
Edgar Cayce: The Sleeping Prophet

Edgar Cayce discovered that he had a psychic gift in 1901 and continued his practice until 1944. Cayce performed over 14,000 psychic readings, the majority of which were for medical purposes, while in a half-sleeping, meditative state, tapping into Universal Consciousness or Intelligence. The diagnoses that he made and the remedies that he recommended were almost 100% effective. Even more amazing is the fact that Cayce had never read a medical textbook nor did he have medical training. His readings covered a wide range of topics, such as religion, ancient civilizations, and predicting the future. His readings were all recorded by a stenographer, classified, and compiled into an enormous body of medical research. Incredibly, this information has not been widely disseminated and used in medical schools. This information is available at the website (http://www.edgarcayce.org) for the Association for Research and Enlightenment (A.R.E.) in Virginia Beach, Va., which was founded by Cayce.

I started my research on Edgar Cayce by reading the book, There is a River by Thomas Sugrue, Then I joined A.R.E. so I could learn more about Cayce's body of work. His work and readings fascinated me.

This whole notion of tapping into Universal Consciousness and performing long distance healing blew my mind. I was a skeptic when I first heard about Cayce's incredible medical accomplishments, but the evidence proving his capabilities was overwhelming.

If you or a loved one has an illness that conventional medicine is not addressing, I encourage you to explore the Cayce readings there may be something there for you. Some of the suggested therapies are exotic and the ingredients not easily acquired. Others, like the castor oil packs, are quite easy to use and have been proven to provide relief. Don't ever let someone tell you that you have an incurable disease until you have turned over every rock and looked for alternative cures. The Cayce case histories provide a source of hope for everyone.

The prescriptions Cayce gave people are akin to the readings that you get from biofeedback devices or radethesia and were designed specifically for the individual who was being treated. As previously mentioned, everyone's energy field is different. (Healing is all about energy fields, so taking a treatment for one patient and applying it to another is not always advisable.) A.R.E has done some correlation work on all of the accumulated Cayce readings and has come up with some standard formulations that seem to work on most people for specific illnesses. But this is a starting point that helps narrow down some of the possible healing options out of 14,000 readings.

Cayce's results speak for themselves. However, if you are motivated to learn and try them out, I encourage you to do so with the aid of a trained physician.

Editor's note:
The concept of Universal Intelligence is very "new age" and foreign to most people. The fact that Edgar Cayce could lie down, go to sleep, and then recite accurate diagnoses and remedies for patients, with no formal medical training, is unbelievable. His patients, in most cases, were people whom he had never met and who, in some cases, were physically halfway around the world from him. Preposterous…right? Having personally read through at least 100 of the case studies I am convinced beyond a shadow of a doubt that energy medicine works. The 14,000 documented Cayce readings are proof.

Examples of the Existence of Universal Intelligence Are Everywhere

Mozart began composing incredibly complex and beautiful symphonies at the age of five. He had no idea where the notes were coming from, he just wrote them down. He astounded and amazed musicians five times his age with his abilities and continues to do so today.

There are child prodigies in many disciplines who have no clue where their ideas, art, or brilliant creations originate. They just "show up." From where?

Albert Einstein, one of the most revered geniuses of all time, proposed the theory of relativity and composition of all matter. He did this without the aid of computers or other high tech apparatus. These concepts just came to him. From where? Universal Intelligence, that's where.

Fellow students in high school and college absolutely astounded me by getting perfect results on a Chemistry examination when they had neither paid attention in class nor studied for it. They just "got it." (I never had this gift.)

Evidence abounds in our world that there is an Intelligence that we can all tap into, if we are resonating at the correct frequency.

Here is a sample Cayce reading 1196–15[1]

This psychic reading given by Edgar Cayce at his home on Arctic Crescent, Virginia Beach, Va., this 24th day of May, 1940, in accordance with request made by the self—Mr. [1196], Associate Member of the Ass"n for Research & Enlightenment, Inc.

PRESENT

Edgar Cayce; Gertrude Cayce, Conductor; Gladys Davis, Steno.

---

1   Cayce reading 1196–15 Virginia Beach, Virginia USA

173 Rich Remedies

READING

Time of Reading 3:45 to 3:55 P.M. Eastern Standard Time...., Alabama.

1. GC: You will give the physical condition of this body at the present time, with suggestions for further corrective measures; answering the questions, as I ask them:

2. EC: Yes, we have the body here; this we have had before.

3. As we find, there has been begun—in part—those suggestions which have been indicated, that WILL bring about the better conditions for this body, if there is the persistent and consistent use of the same.

4. It is indicated by the conditions which arise that there are those disturbances as we have indicated through the gall duct and gall bladder area, as well as the effect that these spasmodic reactions have upon the conditions through the intestinal tract, especially the colon, and the effect that is produced upon the locomotory system.

5. Then, we would continue systematically with those applications that have been suggested; namely: the Castor Oil Packs,—these taken three days in succession for at least an hour each time; followed by the Olive Oil taken internally as indicated.

6. Those injections and the use of the compounds given for the emptying of the gall duct are also helpful. With the combinations, these at times become rather a strenuous activity, and requires that the body rest a great deal during the periods that the Packs are given, of the evenings that these are given.

7. However, if these will be continued, with the leaving off of any

sedative as much as possible, they will prove effective.

8. Take plenty of water at all times.

9. We would take the salts on the days when the Castor Oil Packs are NOT taken,—and when taking same (after the injections that have been indicated), lie upon the right side with a pillow under the body at the liver and gall duct area.

10. As the system is cleansed of these poisons, it will be found well to have one or two colonic irrigations,—once or twice each month,—so long as these treatments are being given; that there may be the poisons eliminated that have accumulated in the alimentary canal, through the activity of these properties on the system, without being reabsorbed in the system by remaining in the intestinal or colon area.

11. Hence we would flush the colon with water, using a little saline (salt) and soda solution in same; this would prove most beneficial, taking away those tendencies for so much weakness and dizziness, and purifying the body better.

12. Be mindful as to the diets,—and keep along those lines that have been heretofore indicated for the body.

13. Ready for questions.

14. (Q) Should I continue to take the tonic after meals also?
(A) This will be very well, IF there is the closer adherence to these applications, in seeing that the salts AND the Packs do not overlap, but come rather consecutively. Do not leave off the Castor Oil Packs!

15. (Q) Is the treatment of Dr. Buresch, German woman doctor, going to cure me?
(A) Not of itself,—else we would not have given these others!

16. (Q) What part of it is the most important?

(A) To keep it up sufficient to drain the gall bladder, and the gall duct, and to keep the poisons so drained out of the system.

16. We are through for the present.

The above sample is representative of thousands of Cayce remedies. Some simple and some very involved, requiring hard-to-find ingredients and very odd combinations of substances. The key is they worked. No surgery was required, punctures, radiation, or any invasive procedures. The cures are effected through resonance and energy. Like all prescriptions, many will work for some, yet be completely ineffective for others.

My Experience

My personal experience has been limited to Cayce's castor oil treatments. My family has used the castor oil packs with good results for treating menstrual cramps, constipation, muscle cramps, indigestion, fever, chills, lower back pain, and dry skin.

Here is the formula for the Castor Oil Pack.[2]

Flannel towel soaked with castor oil (organic, cold pressed). Heat to 120 degrees Fahrenheit. Fold towel and place on abdomen. Be sure that the towel is not too hot! Place a heating pad or hot water bottle over the soaked towel(Place plastic foil under your treated area to catch oil that may soil sheets or clothing. Keep pad in place for one (1) hour. Take one tablespoon of olive oil. Repeat according to Cayce directions.

---

[2] McGarey, William A.. *The Oil That Heals: A Physician's Successes with Castor Oil Treatments.* Virginia Beach: A.R.E. Press, 1993. Pages 26–27.

Castor oil has an energetic resonance, a frequency that promotes healing. Cayce sited over fifty different conditions of illness that would benefit from its use.

Cayce routinely diagnosed and suggested effective cures for people with terminal illnesses who had been written off for dead by their doctors. On several occasions he was arrested for practicing medicine without a license. As it seems with the American medical establishment, "no good deed goes unpunished," especially when you are helping people avoid hospitals and massive medical expenses.

By all accounts, Edgar Cayce was a generous, modest, God-fearing man with a special gift that he shared with people from all walks of life. His legacy and body of work do not receive the recognition that they deserve. There is a huge reservoir of self-healing knowledge available to everyone through A.R.E. which I recommend that you join, so that you, too, can tap into its many natural healing resources.

SECTION 4
TWO THINGS OF IMMENSE IMPORTANCE: WATER AND YOUR MIND

Chapter 18
Water as Healing Medicine

Water is the Soup of Life

Water is magic. It carries energy and possesses many healing qualities that I will discuss here. You could probably start and end this book with just water; it is such an amazing healing, life sustaining substance.

Our very survival here on this planet depends on water. Life on Earth cannot be sustained without water. All human civilization is based on ready access to water. Seventy percent of our bodies are made up of water. Ten days without water and you will die! If you are an adult of normal weight, you can live up to 70 days without food, or seven times longer than you can without water. Next to oxygen, water is the most important substance that you need for survival and one of the most overlooked nutritional elements in the daily diet. You can argue that water is more important than oxygen since a lot of our oxygen comes from water (H2O).

Soda pop, caffeinated drinks, milk, and sports drinks have been substituted for water in the daily American diet. You may argue that all of these liquids contain some water, but consuming them is not the same as drinking a pure glass of water. In some cases, even if you are drinking water by itself, it has been contaminated with chemicals and bacteria in our municipal water systems.

Can you image the impact that you can have on your health by improving the component that makes up 70% of your physical body? That's a very high percentage of the physical "you" we're talking about here! There are energetic and spiritual aspects to water that I discovered while writing this book.

When I first wrote this chapter I was unaware of Masuru Emoto's inspiring book *The Hidden Messages in Water*. After reading his book, and seeing his pictures of water crystals, I have an even greater appreciation and respect for water. As a result, I changed the beginning of this chapter to briefly acknowledge his wonderful discoveries. Initially I had focused on the obvious nutritional benefits of water, but then I realized there are much broader energetic benefits.

If you've made it this far in this book, you'd be disappointed if I did not offer some esoteric angle on water's energetic properties. How it resonates according to different frequencies that come from sounds, words, emotions, photos, and all energetic sources. Wouldn't you? Well of course I won't disappoint you.

Emoto discovered, through special magnified photographic techniques, that water, when frozen, forms crystals that change shape when exposed to certain vibrations, including thoughts, prayers, intentions, music, and written or spoken words, and pollution. (No crystals were detected in any polluted water he tested.) His photographs have been scientifically validated and are a "must see".

Other interesting things that he discovered are:
- Water is a transporter of energy
- Water has the ability to copy and memorize information
- Water circulates around the globe and picks up everything it passes
- Water crystals react to music, emotions, photos, prayers, and words (See Emoto's pictures for proof)
- Love and gratitude form the most beautiful water crystals
- Water is sensitive to frequencies and mirrors the world
- Water resonates with Ki, your life energy.

181 Rich Remedies

On several occasions Emoto observed miraculous things with water. In one such encounter, he observed Houki Kato, a Shinto priest of the Shingon Sect; repeat a prayer at the Fujiwara dam lake in Japan. (Water in the lake had stagnated and was polluted before the prayer.) The energy from the prayers purified the water in the lake, and changed the crystal structure. This determination was based on actual before and after measurements that were taken.[3] True story.

So what is the relevance and significance of this interesting and esoteric information from Masuru Emoto on water, you ask?

I find Emoto's work relevant to the subject of healing on all levels. The physical changes occurring in water as the result of human intentions, expressions and sounds are the same as those made on you and me at a deep molecular level. Words, music, sounds, vibrations all resonate into the body, beyond a level that I ever comprehended and directly into your personal body water. So it's not just your brain and senses that are being affected by your experiences, but also your personal body water. Seventy percent of your physical body is feeling and absorbing these energetic impressions because you are mostly water. I think this is profound. I never looked at it this way. It's something to think about. If you see his photos, you'll know what I mean.

Now, on to the less mind-bending but equally important health aspects of water.

Water is the medium for life. Since the body is comprised of 70% water, it is critical that you are drinking a lot of water of high quality and purity. With our current municipal water systems, this is extremely challenging since chlorine, fluoride, bacteria, sludge, and other what-not is sometimes flowing through the pipes. There is some variability between different municipal water systems' water quality, so it is advisable to filter your water no matter where you are.

---

2 Emoto, Masaru. *Messages from Water.* Hillsboro, Ore.: Beyond Words Publishing, Inc., 1999

In this section of the chapter I will discuss water consumption guidelines, filters, and other fun facts. If you do nothing but consume pure, healthy water in the recommended quantities, you are making huge strides towards improving your health. This is the easiest thing to do in this book.

It is recommended that you consume one-half your body weight in ounces of pure water each day. On average this works out to be 8 ounces, 8 times per day. (For a person weighing 150 lbs, 75 ounces of water should be consumed.) This seems like a lot, but your body needs this. There are some who suggest that we consume too much water, placing a strain on the digestive system. Personally, I subscribe to the rule of consuming more, not less, water for proper hydration.

Here is the recommended minimum pure water consumption per day. More may be required if you are sick, dehydrated, or physically exerting yourself.

Body weight	Ounces per day	8 oz glasses per day
50 lbs or less	25	3
100 lbs	50	6.25
150 lbs	75	9.3
200 lbs	100	12.5

This water consumption guideline is so obvious and self-evident, yet few people actually follow it. Just watch what they drink on any given day and you'll see.

Drinking healthy water is the most important step towards maintaining good health; one that everyone can and should take. It is fundamental to your survival, and requires minimal sacrifice, or change to your routine, unless you do not presently drink water. Many people drink soda pop and other beverages instead of water.

Drinking clean, healthy water may be a big step for some people, but it is a necessary one.

Ionized Water

As discussed earlier, high pH fluids and foods help fight disease and reverse the condition known as acidosis.

Ionized water is water that has a negative charge or is ionized. Acting as an anti-oxidant, it reduces oxidation or aging in the body. On the other hand, processed foods and beverages, having a positive charge, oxidize, and cause aging. (I replaced our standard water filter with a water ionizer in order to clean and ionize our water in an effort to lower our collective family pH, thus offsetting the junk food that still finds its way into our cupboard.)

A simple example of how pH works is the treatment used for cleaning swimming pools of clouds of algae. When the pH gets low, algae forms turning the water green and cloudy. Eventually, the pool becomes unfit for bathing due to its polluted, acidic state. The same thing happens with your bodly fluids. When your body pH gets low, you attract molds, bacteria, yeast, and other disease-causing toxins. Fostering high pH with lots of ionized water is a great disease prevention tool.

Here is a quote I offer from an expert in ionized water's healing effects:

"The anti oxidant water contains an abundance of ionic calcium. This ionic calcium helps in the "burn off" process. By drinking antioxidant water, it provides sufficient minerals for our body. As a result we do not need to watch our diet to stay slim. Hence, antioxidant water is the savior for those suffering from obesity and many other adult diseases, providing good assistance in enhancing good health."

— Professor Hatori Tasutaroo,
The Use of Ionized Water in Treating Acidosis[1]

Agricultural, residential, and industrial pollution have rendered much of our drinking water toxic. In my neighborhood in Austin, we received letters from the local municipal water department that we have exceeded the maximum containment of trihalomethyanes (TTHMs), a group of volatile organic compounds that are formed when chlorine (which is added to the water during treatment pro¬cess for disinfection) reacts with naturally-occurring organic matter in the water. TTHMs can cause liver and kidney damage and, in some cases, cancer. Chlorine is a common chemical used in water treatment so chances are that you are being exposed to this poison. Our water originates in the Texas hill country lakes which flow into the upper Colorado River, then through Lake Travis and, ultimately Lake Austin. It's got to be good, right?

Fluoride, once promoted as a healthy additive to protect against tooth decay, was added to municipal drinking supplies. Fluoride is toxic when consumed in large quantities and is now being banned by many municipal water authorities. Whoever owned the fluoride chemical production companies in the 1950s really suckered the US health officials, bribed them or both. Fluoride is not meant for human consumption. Get a filter that removes this poison from your water. Don't be fooled by the "experts" who tell you fluoride is good for you. It isn't.

Drinking bottled water is not always a guarantee that you are drinking pure water. Some bottled water is filtered, minimally processed tap water that has a pH between 4 to 6 which is acidic. Sometimes you will get a plastic after-taste which suggests to me that you're getting some plastic olefins as an extra bonus. The pack¬aging and labeling will lead you to believe that you are getting something special, but in some cases, you'd be better off saving the dollar and walking over to the kitchen tap for a drink. Municipal water by law needs to have a pH of 7.0. There are no regulations on pH within the bottled water industry

---

3   Tasutaroo, Hatori PhD, *The Use of Ionized Water in Treating Acidosis, Akajuiiji Blood Center, Yokahama Hospital, Faitama District, Japan*

My Experience

Everybody seems to at least acknowledge the fact that you need pure water but, like avoiding excess sugar and fast food, few of us consciously follow the 8 glasses a day rule. I emphasize pure water.

When I lived in Pennsylvania there were natural springs by the side of the road where you could gather water. People, including me would line up with 12 gallon jugs to collect this supposedly health-giving spring water. After a few years the taps on the natural springs were shut down due to bacterial contamination as a result of run-off from nearby septic systems and pastures where livestock were grazing. (Never assume that any water is pure and clean, not even in the countryside where there aren't lots of people and industry to pollute the water.)

At our home in the country, we had a deep well that had been drilled 60 feet below ground, to insure a steady flow during draughts and cleanliness. The water, we discovered, was acidic, turning our sinks and basins green from the copper pipe that it was dissolving. (It also turned my wife's blond hair green.) I was quite certain that our internal health was suffering from the acidic water, so we switched to the delivery of bottled spring water. We could not wait to move to a development with clean municipal tap water. Our "healthy" country well water was anything but healthy.

Unfortunately, what I have discovered is that most sources of water, including expensive bottled water, contain some level of contamination and tend to be acidic. The plastic, bottled water has plastic in it. I still drink bottled water when nothing else is available, but I do not buy it by the case like I used to. Tap water is better for you, if you have a filter.

I recommend that you invest in a water purification system for your house or, at a minimum, your kitchen sink. Filtration systems can cost as little as $100, eliminating the need to buy cases or jugs of bottled spring water. My first water purifier delivered 1000 gallons of pure, filtered water before the filter needed replacing. The water tastes great, is free of most contaminants, costs pennies on the dollar, is convenient, and leverages the money that I am already paying to the water company.

There is some debate amongst experts as to the true healing effects of Ionized water. I can only speak from my personal experience and say that I feel it is beneficial. Some of the benefits attributed to Inonized water are the following:

- Ionized water is a powerful antioxidant
- It provides increased oxygen and free radical scavengers
- It's alkalinity balances your body pH
- It's a powerful detoxifier and superior hydrator

Ionized water is worth the investment for your family's health. Consuming pure, toxin-free water will deliver immediate health benefits with minimal effort. What you can't see in your water, can potentially make you sick.

Another measure that I take is placing a gallon jug of water one foot away from a full spectrum light for thirty minutes. Dr. Hazel Parcels experimented with the use of full-spectrum lighting as a means of purifying water with excellent results. I don't completely understand how the light waves purify the water, but I use it. Try it out. For the cost of a $10 full spectrum light bulb you may be getting purer water. A water store here in Austin is using this light method as part of a reverse osmosis filtering system, to purify water that it has for sale, so there is probably some benefit. By the way, reverse osmosis water is on the more acidic side of the alkaline scale so it is pure, but higher in acid than ionized water.

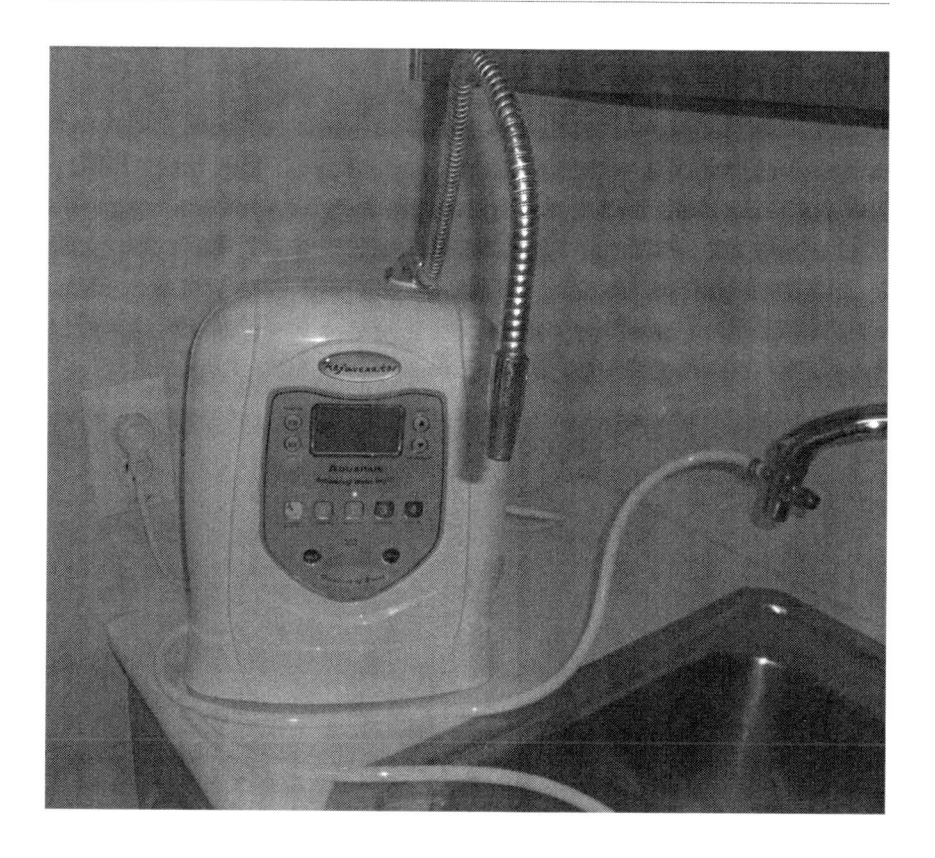

This is the water Ionizer that I use. Note that it discharges alkaline water out of the stainless steel faucet for internal use and acidic water for external use.

EM•X® Ceramics in Water

High temperature ceramics treated with EM™ have been used to condition and treat water. The EM™ "activates water by making its molecular clusters smaller" according to product literature. The EM•X® Ceramics product description also says "7 micron particles are effective at creating spin in water", conditioning it. This is a new discovery that will be researched further and discussed in the sequel to this book.

Other healing properties of water

In nature, water provides all sorts of subtle healing effects. The sound and movement of a waterfall calms and relaxes. The water falling and colliding with rocks, vaporizes, creating oxygen and negative ions which are health-giving. Crashing ocean waves have the same hypnotic as well as ionizing effect. So the next time you are sitting by a waterfall or crashing waves, know that, while you are enjoying the view, you are getting a healthy dose of negative ions.

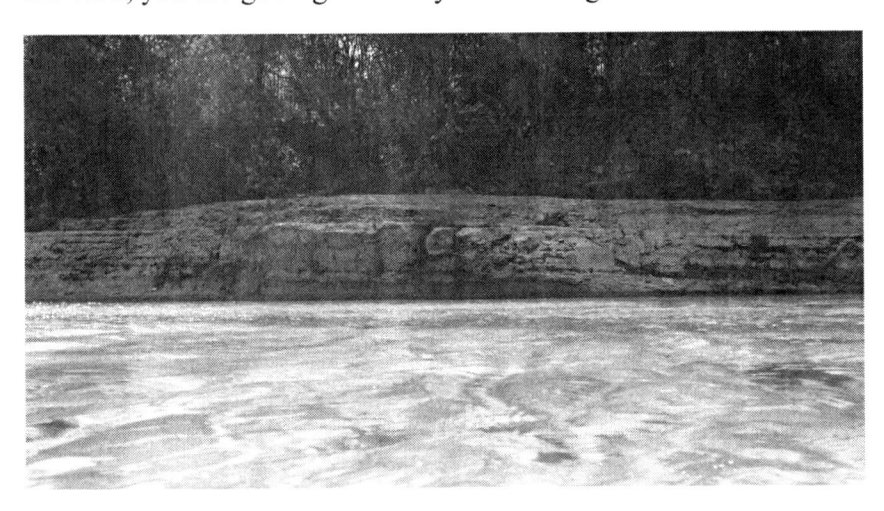

Barton Springs Pool in the City of Austin is a healing water place. The spring is fed by the Edwards Aquifer, a natural, underground reservoir. It flows underground through the limestone caverns of the Texas Hill Country from Kyle to Austin where it spills into the Lady Bird Lake (Colorado River) at the end of its journey. Barton Springs was a sacred place for Native Americans and remains so today for many of us in Austin.

Reflecting pools, fountains, ponds, and man-made lakes are landscape designs that feature water as a focal point, creating beautiful, natural backdrops and living spaces. People pay top dollar for oceanfront, lakefront, riverfront, and creek front property.

What is it that attracts us to water? We are water.

Chapter 19
The Mind/Body Connection

"I have seen chronic illnesses alleviated in the bodies of patients whose minds are at peace. Some people have noted energy shifts when insights and understandings emerge. The mind and body are so intimately connected that healing one heals the other."
— Dr. Brian Weisse, Same Soul, Many Bodies.[2]

A simplistic diagram of an undulating line was drawn on the black board. The line was a series of smoothed semi circles (sine waves) flowing one after the other. This simple illustration was drawn on a blackboard by a Native American Apache healer, William Two Feather during a Native American "Drum Washing" healing class that I attended.[3] According to Two Feather, nature has a rhythm of its own that when honored, promotes harmony and healing. When disrupted by negative energy, destructive human emotions, actions, creations, or any "bad vibrations" creates chaos and nature's flow is disrupted. The good energy and natural order of things becomes disrupted. If you have any connection with nature you know this to be true.

An interesting aside is that William Two Feather has been on a teaching pilgrimage around the world to disseminate the Native American healing traditions that were kept secret from nontribal

---

2   Weisse, Brian L. *Same Soul, Many Bodies.* New York, NY: Simon and Shuster, 2004. Page 171.

3   *Two Feather, William, Apache Medicine Man, Drum Washing Instruction,* Austin, Texas. March 10–11, 2007

members until the Harmonic Convergence, August 17, 1987. When I heard this I was surprised and delighted that the Harmonic Convergence had a greater significance than just a bunch of New Agers doing a line dance around Stone Henge. These Native American Healing Traditions that are being revealed for the first time in history are phenomenal.

In his travels, William has observed that all of the natural healing traditions around the world contain the same concepts and basic Spiritual practices. It's called the Truth. The truth is the same no matter where you go in the world. It makes sense. Read all of the good religious texts and they are all saying the same thing. Truth—it's the same everywhere.

It has taken me years of scratching my head to figure out exactly what this is all about. It is a very simple concept, creating a frequency match with nature or Spirit. I sure haven't mastered it, but at least I understand the end game and have the ability to work on myself. Buddhist monks spend decades meditating to get to this state of consciousness and oneness with the Spirit, so I don't feel too bad that my level of "clarity" is rather modest at this time. But I consciously work on this every day. Right now I don't have a year to take off to meditate in silence, which is one thing monks do, to get in touch with their inner self.

"Self Healing" is a process of getting your energy to match the frequencies (thoughts, feelings, emotions) in your mind/body in a smooth, flowing way, synching up with Spirit. This is accomplished by thinking, feeling, and visualizing positive thoughts and emotions (Love). Actually "Being Love."

My goal here is not to sound like some pious guru. I am not pious and I'm certainly not a guru. What I am saying is that this concept of "being love" is contained in every enlightened spiritual tradition in the world. It is the single thread that runs universally through all belief systems, so it is worthy of your consideration as it relates to healing.

Prayer, meditation, and visualization are three common practices used to promote self-healing. Living your life by the Golden Rule; treat people and all things the way you wish to be treated, is also a fundamental component.

This kernel of truth is contained in every worthwhile religious text that has ever been written, yet for some reason few of us can put this basic natural concept into practice on a consistent basis including this author. Some philosophers blame our inability to attain this unity of mind and spirit on the human ego which is never satisfied with what is and is always seeking more.

The concept of a Mind/Body/Spirit connection may sound "Pollyannaish," feel-good, and new age, but it's absolutely true and the healing effects of an enlightened consciousness are fully supported by science. Read any of the numerous books on quantum physics and you will see that what I am saying is true. For a good introduction to quantum physics, read *What the Bleep Do We Know? Discovering the Endless possibilities for Altering Your Everyday Reality.*[1] The book supports the notion that you create your reality. A peaceful, centered consciousness creates a peaceful, healthy, happy life.

All of this relates directly to the oldest, yet newest, concept on the planet, the Law of Attraction. In a spiritual context, it is the rule that states "you reap what you sow," or you become what you think about in your mind all day long. Our minds are powerful energy forces, magnets with incomprehensible strength creating and attracting everything you see into your life. It (your mind) molds your life experiences and health according to the way that you think every second of every day.

If you do not deliberately manage your thoughts (frequencies) in a positive way, your body will produce chemicals, like cortisol and adrenalin that will literally poison you. With negative thinking you will also produce electrical blockages that will result in "short

---

1 Arntz, William, Betsy Chasse, and Mark Vincente. *What the Bleep Do We Know!?: Discovering the endless possibilities for altering your everyday reality.* Deerfield Beach, Fla: Health Communications, Inc., 2005.

circuits" in your meridians that will, in turn, affect the connected organs and tissues. Negative thoughts such as fear, envy, hate, and jealousy are acid-producing and can actually lower the pH of your body. As discussed in several previous chapters, acidosis is one of the fundamental causes of cell degeneration in the body, just like acidic foods that we eat. Thoughts are things, like food, believe it or not.

All physical manifestations start in your mind. Our task is to continuously, consciously manage our thoughts in a positive way all day long. Keep that little area of the Universe, the "You" clean, tidy, and uncluttered of mental debris. Health is yours! Your 220 trillion cells are buzzing with everything you feed them, including your thoughts. The whole system: mind, body, and soul are interconnected. Be vigilant as to what you allow to occupy your mind, in the same way you need to watch what you're eating.

This basic truth about the mind/body connection has been known for centuries. The Buddhists call the "good, positive" frequency matching satori or bliss. It's when your mind and body are synchronized with the rhythmic patterns of Spirit and nature. Another term for this synchronization is "entrainment." Eastern religions and indigenous people around the world have known and practiced religious rituals that bring them into these blissful states since the beginning of time. All of our great spiritual leaders attained these heightened states of consciousness. However, these practices have somehow been lost to many of us in the West, although we are now gradually rediscovering them. This book is my small attempt to bring a higher level of consciousness and awareness back to those of us who have forgotten. I say forgotten because all of us know what the truth is at a deep level. It's just been buried by all of our modern distractions and preoccupations.

Evidence of an awakening taking place in conventional medicine can be seen in certain enlightened cancer hospitals. Cancer therapy in these hospitals is focusing a lot of attention on the patient's mental, emotional, and spiritual state to effectively reverse the disease, in combination with conventional therapies like chemo therapy, radiation, and surgery. Patients are being treated as "whole beings" instead of as just cancer sufferers.

The pathology of thoughts

An interesting concept that supports this mind/ body / spirit concept is the work done separately by Bernie Siegel, MD and Louise Hay. They both discovered a mental and physiological phenomenon they refer to as "target organs."[2] The concept is that certain fears and emotions created in the mind actually target specific organs of the body, causing diseases. The pathology (source of diseases) can be traced, in part, to specific thought patterns that people engage in on a consistent, predictable basis. Louise Hay devotes a whole section of her book, *You Can Heal Your Life*, to specific thought/ disease correlations.

This was very revealing to me and strongly motivated me to watch what I say and think. If you want to increase the probability of being healthy, keep track of what you're thinking and then raise the quality or the frequency (vibration) of your thoughts. Raise your thought patterns to positive, optimistic, and upbeat. Generate your own good vibes. This is another remedy that costs you nothing!

> *"The body knows only what the mind tells it."*
> — David Bohm, PhD

---

2 Siegel, Bernie, MD, Love, Medicine & Miracles:New York, NY.Harper & Row Publishers, 1986, Page 90.

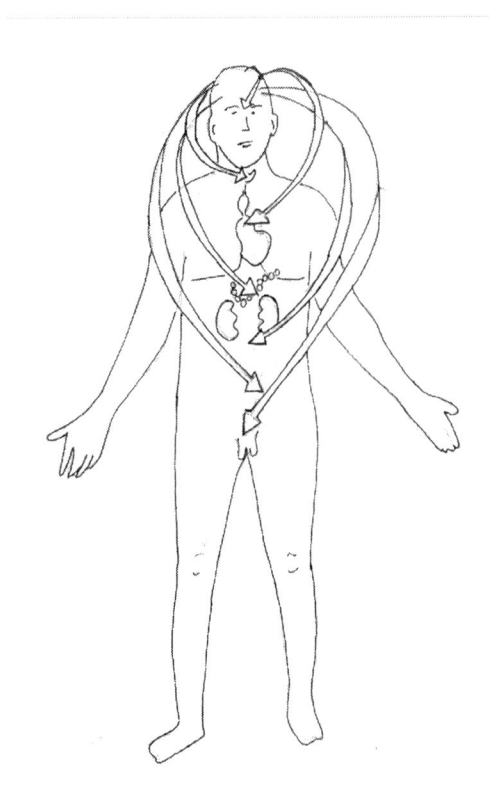

Here's a simple illustration:

In a disease state, we sensitize the target organs in our body with a form of negative biofeedback, a fancy term for the mind energetically creating disease in your body.

"Target organs", parts of the body with special significance to the conflicts or losses in a person's life, are the most likely areas for disease to take root. Franz Alexander, the father of psychosomatic medicine, recognized this over 40 years ago when he wrote: "there is much evidence that, just as certain pathological microorganisms have a specific affinity for certain organs, so also certain emotional conflicts possess specificities and accordingly tend to afflict certain internal organs."[3]

Rich Remedies

Attitude was recognized as a source of illness in many of Edgar Cayce's diagnosis. Cayce, the great American psychic and diagnostician often recommended that fixing a bad attitude is a way to help cure a disease. "No one can hate his neighbor and not have stomach or liver trouble. No one can be jealous and allow anger of same and not have upset digestion or heart disorder." (Edgar Cayce reading 4021-1)

Emotional healing on the surface sounds simple and it is really easy to write about. Now try doing it! I'm in a constant state of ridding myself of this embedded mental junk, on a daily basis, it never stops. Just when I think it's gone, some emotional wart rears its ugly head. It takes practice. In my case, life has been relatively easy. For those of you who have had a tough road in life with a lot of mental and physical abuse, disposing of bad memories can be a difficult, lengthy task indeed.

There are two metaphors I use to explain mental debris that accumulates in the mind which cause illness if you don't consciously work at clearing it. This debris is a combination of stress, past traumas, disappointments, fears, personal affronts, phobias, and useless tribal beliefs that are, in many cases, undetected by the conscious mind but slush around in your unconscious mind. The river and old house metaphors are how I explain the concealed mental crud that often lies dormant and needs clearing.

A river flows down stream carrying particles of sediment, depositing them along the river bottom. Years of living and experiences are layered like sediment in the river one on top of the other. Each successive emotion covers up the one before it or we use coping mechanisms to ignore them so they get buried deeper, but never go away. This also happens in your body with physical diseases that are masked, but sometimes not cured, by medicine. They remain dormant waiting for emotional stress or the immune

---

3   Siegel, Bernie, MD, Love, Medicine & Miracles:New York, NY.Harper & Row Publishers, 1986. Page 90.

system to weaken so they can re-emerge.

As I went through the Asyra diagnostic process (described in Chapter 11. Biomagnetic Screening, new disease signatures showed up on my screening report as old ones disappeared, even after weeks of nutritional therapy and cleansing.

A "signature" is a small trace or frequency that is picked up by the Asyra device indicating the presence of a virus, bacteria, or even an emotion issue. As discussed earlier, every organism emits its own, unique energy frequency.

If you work long enough at cleansing and nutritional therapy, you will eventually clear all the dormant dis-ease from your body. It's like scraping the paint off of a 200 year old colonial-era house that has had many owners. Each successive occupant paints the original wood a different color. Some are awful; others are tasteful. The layers cover up the beautiful natural wood that needed no embellishment in the first place, like your true self or spirit. We cover or corrupt our pure spirit with layers of fear and anger concealing the basic goodness that is Source.

In the example of the old house, it sometimes takes scraping ten layers of paint before finding the original, beautiful wood below. When you get down to the original wood, you sand it, stain it and varnish it so it looks like it did originally. Beautiful, natural grain wood. The restoration is hard, time consuming work. But the end result is beautiful. The same goes for cleansing a life's worth of memories from your subconscious mind! This layer clearing is what we need to do to completely and thoroughly heal ourselves. That's my opinion. What's yours?

Prayer

Having excused myself from regular church attendance for some of my adult life, it seems odd to me that prayer finds its way into my book. Hypocrisy you say? Actually, the forced march as a youth in the Catholic Church never diminished my faith in the power of prayer. The people running the Church sometimes disillusioned me, but the core teachings that were good never left me. If you take the corrupting influences of people out of religion, you are usually left with very good and useful teachings to manage our spiritual lives.

A thought leader on the mind/body/spirit connection as it pertains to the power of prayer is Dr. Norman Shealy. In the book, co-authored with Dawson Church PhD, Soul Medicine, there are several findings relevant to a discussion of nonphysical things that direct your physical being. Prayer is one of them. Shealy and Church have documented many case studies as proof that spiritual practice and beliefs have a marked influence on longevity and health. There is a spiritual dimension to healing that cannot be denied. There is a God.

In Soul Medicine they discuss a University of Texas Medical School Study led by Thomas Oxman that found that a patient's religious and spiritual beliefs positively impacted their healing from heart surgery. The study found that: "patients who possessed a large and deep social network, or were devoted to their religious or spiritual practice, exhibited just one seventh the mortality rate of those that did not."[4] Another study showed that death and re-hospitalization rates were 30% lower for patients who were prayed for by others. Thirty percent is statistically significant and cannot be chalked up to coincidence. Prayer works.

In Dr. Larry Dossey's book, Reinventing Medicine, there are the results of a number of studies showing that among heart patients, those who were prayed for had better clinical outcomes than those who had medical therapy alone. A similar case showed that AIDS patients who were being prayed for experienced fewer and less severe AIDS-related illnesses.[5]

---

4   Shealy, Norman,. and Dawson Church. Soul Medicine: Awakening Your Inner Blueprint for Abundant Health and Energy. Santa Rosa, Cal.: Elite Books, 2006. Page 18.

5   Weisse, Brian L. Same Soul, Many Bodies. New York, NY: Simon and Shuster, 2004. Page 53.

Past Life Regression Therapy

The last and final frontier that I will touch on, since it involves the mind/body/ spirit connection, is past lives and their impact on your present life. I wasn't going to go into these relatively uncharted waters, but I want to share some interesting things that I found. My mind was opened to the possibility that there may be some validity to the concept of carrying past life trauma and illness with you into this life and then curing it. There are illnesses that defy curing by typical holistic and allopathic healing practices because the source of the illness is deep inside your Soul. These are the unexplainable diseases that defy all healing techniques.

This, I promise you, will be a short chapter as I risk being committed to a sanitarium and getting funny looks from the neighbors and co-workers for this section of my book. (Actually, I'm already toast with the neighbors and co-workers so all I'm really worried about now are the dudes in the white truck with white suits, and the psychotropic drug drip.)

"Past life regression therapy" is an area of medical practice known as parapsychology which deals with "paranormal behavior", or spiritual aspects of a person's psyche.

Believe me, this is hard for me to swallow, but there are multiple doctors with documented clinical cases of patients reporting things from past lives that they could not possibly have known had they not actually been there, in another lifetime, to witness and experience them. There are cases of people reciting ancient documents that they had never seen, speaking foreign languages that they were never taught, describing in vivid details places that they never visited, and recalling all manner of details beyond the scope of their present life experiences. This is viewed by skeptics as science fiction, but through my research I have come to believe it's very real. I have very limited experience with parapsychology and will refer you, as always, to documented sources and experts in the field. If you're interested in past life regression, here are a few tidbits to whet your

Rich Remedies

appetite for further inquiry.

For me the evidence that past life impacts this life is in the work of Michael Newton, PhD, and Brian Weiss, MD, two highly degreed and trained medical professionals who have witnessed first-hand the past life healing phenomenon. That is, your eternal Soul getting in touch with past life experiences that, in some cases, occurred thousands of years ago and affect your present mind and body.

In *Many Lives Many Masters* by Brian Weiss, MD, a patient named Catherine experienced deep fears of water, choking, airplanes, the dark, and dying. They were so strong that she suffered from nightmares which negatively impacted every aspect of her life. She was referred to Dr. Weiss for psychological counseling.[6]

Dr. Weiss, a graduate of Columbia University and Yale University of Medicine, was classically trained in the scientific method and conventional medical therapies. He became a psychiatrist and head of the psychiatry department at a hospital in Miami, Fla. Here Dr. Weiss encountered his patient Catherine, who changed his life and beliefs forever about reincarnation and the effect that past lives have on our present condition.

In summary, Dr. Weiss began past life regression therapy on Catherine, a process that involves hypnotizing a patient into a trance-like state, so that they can uncover chronic phobias from which they suffer and resolve them.

Catherine's initial counseling followed the standard psychological interview and discussion method of childhood memories and life experiences. After a year's worth of conventional counseling, Catherine's condition continued to worsen. On a trip to Chicago, she went to an Egyptian exhibit and began to describe details of ancient Egyptian civilization to the museum guide. She had no previous training in or knowledge of this culture. She reported this odd occurrence to Dr. Weiss who decided to use hypnotherapy to see

---

6   Weiss, Brian L., *"Many Lives, Many Masters".New York, NY: Simon and Shuster.1988. Pages 27–28.*

if there was some deeper meaning to Catherine's bizarre recollection of ancient Egyptian culture. The hypnotherapy uncovered details of multiple past lives starting in Egypt in 1863 BC, Greece in 1568 BC, The Netherlands in 1473 AD, Europe in 1756 AD, and multiple other places and times. In each circumstance she had vivid recall of the details of that life.

Initially, Dr. Weiss was not certain if Catherine was reciting her own fictitious fantasies or if her recollections were, in fact, real. Several incidents convinced him that she was expressing actual details of her own past lives. She also told Dr. Weisse intimate details regarding the life and death of Dr. Weiss' baby daughter, who died one year after she was born. There was no way, in Wess' opinion that she would have known any of the details that she revealed without some deep spiritual connection to the other side. There are a series of fascinating stories about Catherine and many other patients that are documented in Many Lives Many Masters, that will change your mind about reincarnation and past life regression therapy if you're interested – or at least get you thinking in a new way.

Another book that provides some interesting reading on the Spiritual aspects of the human healing experience is Journey of Souls: Case Studies of Life between Lives by Michael Newton, PhD.

I know the concept of using past lives for healing sounds absurd to most people – unless you believe in reincarnation, in which case this is all very real. I would not have included this here if there were not documented, independently verified, clinical evidence, and there had not been witnesses to back up the stories. Believe it if you can. Reincarnation was part of both the Old and New Testaments. In A.D. 325 the Roman emperor Constantine the Great, had references to reincarnation deleted from the New Testament texts. The Second Council of Constantinople, A.D. 553, confirmed this action declaring the concept heresy.[7]

---

7   Weiss, Brian L., "Many Lives, Many Masters".New York, NY: Simon and Shuster.1988. Page 36.

My Experience

Past life regression therapy really fascinates me. I actually tried this twice while doing my research for this book; it totally weirded me out. I'm not sure if during my therapy I was fabricating the stories that came into my mind while being hypnotized, free associating or just saying what entered my mind because it was there. Was this all a movie created in my imagination? Maybe. Was I really seeing my past lives? I don't know. I can tell you I was sufficiently freaked out to limit my therapy sessions to just two. Maybe I'll go back some day.

If I get a chronic illness that confounds me and my health coach, you can bet I'll be back on that couch in a heartbeat. There is definitely merit to past life regression therapy based on all that I have read on the subject, my limited personal experience notwithstanding. For now I will chalk up my two sessions as an exercise to further medical science according to me. Mind expansion is a good thing. I think. The mind/body/spirit link is most definitely a reality, I think there's a lot of work involved in reaching higher states of consciousness where you can use the tremendous powers of your mind. Very often the road to getting the required consciousness involves a serious illness. Sickness forces us into actions that we might not otherwise consider because we are comfortable and preoccupied with everyday living. There's nothing like sickness to wake you up from an unconscious stupor. Illness sometimes drains enough of the ego so that we can more clearly see what is required to repair our health and spirit.

> **In reflecting on the things that I have been able to treat myself, like asthma, allergies, stomach ulcer, and cholesterol, there was most definitely a mental stress component involved. Natural remedies, along with stress management, enabled me to heal these things.**

SECTION 5
BACKGROUND INFORMATION

Chapter 20
My Story
(How "Joe Six pack" got into natural healing)

The Quack, the Hippie and the Refugee

As one of eight children (number 5) born January 16, 1957, I guess I can be considered a late-stage "baby boomer." Raised as a middleclass, Catholic American kid growing up in the 1960s, I was exposed to mainstream, conservative attitudes in politics, religion and healthcare. We ate ham on Easter, fish sticks with macaroni and cheese on Fridays during Lent (meat forbidden) and a generally healthy American diet. Meat and potatoes with some greens on the side and I ate allot of candy and drank prodigious amounts of sugared soda pop. My parents paid their taxes, obeyed the laws, voted Republican and went to church on Sundays and every Catholic holy day. We were a pretty average, conventional American family. I grew up in an area called the "Main Line" in the western suburbs of Philadelphia, Pennsylvania. The suburbs of Philadelphia were developed along the "Main Line" of the Pennsylvania Railroad tracks.

From the time I was a small child, I was frightened of doctors. I had rotting teeth extracted when I was only two years old and vaccinations and booster shots throughout the early years that were painful to receive and hurt for days. Also, as a young tike, my tonsils and adenoids were removed. Some modern theory suggests that extracting my tonsils and adenoids compromised my immune system. At that time, and even now, this was accepted as good medical practice.

My teeth were always bad as a child. It was something I was born with and my sugar cravings aggravated this condition. I always had many cavities. In any case, like many people, I developed a phobia for hospitals and doctors at a very young age that continues to this present day. In part, I attribute my obsession with natural healing to this long standing fear and my aversion to losing control of my body.

As a child I also viewed non-mainstream medicine with suspicion and humor in my home town of Ardmore, Pa, in the 1970's.. There was a natural health food store. The old woman who ran the place was heavy, had a peculiar odor and a lazy eye. The eye was canted to the side so she could work the cash register and watch the door at the same time. She had a built-in security camera going. A real innovator. Not a picture of good health nor the best spokes model for health food and nutrition. I used to associate "health food" with peculiar, odd people since my first impressions were colored by the Ardmore Health Food Store operators and others I saw buying the strange potions that were sold at the store.

Her male colleague was equally "unique". He was tall, balding, and sickly skinny, as some health enthusiasts often appear. They were an interesting combination: evangelical Christians, vegetarians, and members of the John Birch Society, a radical, rightwing, organization, Ultra right wing granola champers. You don't find many of them around!

The store had radical right wing newsletters and periodicals mixed with quirky back to nature brochures. It seemed like quite a contrast to me. Into nature, healing, and separation all at one time. I couldn't figure them out and they colored my early impression of natural healing and natural foods. I think the attitude I formed in my youth towards the natural health industry and practitioners is very common among people in the US. This attitude is quickly changing as people wake up and stores like Whole Foods Market and even

Wal-Mart take natural healing products to the mainstream.

An incident that further colored my impression of the health food store that still makes me laugh today was the time my friend Tom tried to buy rubbers at the Ardmore Health food store.

Tom knew that I frequented the store and asked me if they sold rubbers (prophylactics) there. I told him that he had to go to Morris Drugs, two doors down from the health food store. He either did not understand me or was not listening. He went into the health food store and asked the holy roller, right wing prudes for a box of rubbers He had no idea of their religious/ political sensitivities or their quirkiness.

The old woman behind the counter freaked out on poor Tom. "Rubbers? Vatt do you mean by rubbers young man? Oh, prophylactics? Is Datt vat you are looking for in here? "She stammered in her thick, Eastern European accent, "We don't sell rubbers. Young man, you should be ashamed of yourself buying rubbers." Tom got completely reamed out by the store owners. Funny. We still laugh about this incident. He dared to soil their sacred ground with his simple, not-so-innocent pubescent request. Tom still carries the scars from that teenage humiliation to this day. He steers clear of health food and health food stores. I have recommended him to a syntonic optometrist for post traumatic stress disorder therapy. He refuses to comply with my recommendation, instead choosing to suffer nightmares to this day.

Another early mind-shaping negative association with alternative healing was a therapist, who lived and worked down the street from my house, who had a car I liked. He owned and drove a mint condition 1960 Studebaker Golden Hawk which, I admired from afar every day I passed his driveway. I grew up a car nut and knew a nice set of wheels when I saw one. The therapist was a chiropractor. I used to ask about the therapist with the hot car, and my elders would tell me that he is a chiropractor, which meant he was a "quack doctor". This was said repeatedly with such conviction that I believed "chiropractor" and "quack" were the same word. Now I know different, but this illustrates how our attitudes are shaped from an early age on alternative medicine. There is a reason that some of us believe alternative medicine is "witchcraft", but will discuss this in the last chapter of this book.

So from early on, like most people, I was conditioned by experience and those around me to suspect and doubt natural food and alternative medicine. So, how did I change? What were my epiphanies?

"The Quack"

I attended "tiny Widener College" as the announcer Howard Cosell would say on ABC Monday Night Football in the early days of that weekly sports broadcast.

I have never heard another televised reference to my alma mater. It was the only college I could get into and that admission was on academic probation. You see, I was a real whiz kid in high school. My focus at this time in my life was on girls, keeping gas in my car and other non-productive activities that I won't cover here since I have teenage children. (I need to maintain my patina and illusion of moral perfection for their benefit.)

Widener had a decent Division 3 football program and graduated All-Pro offensive center Joe Fields of the New York Jets and punt/kickoff return specialist Billy "White Shoes" Johnson, of the Houston Oilers. Other than these fun facts there is not much to say about Widener. I am grateful that they took me off the streets of Philadelphia and gave me a place to hang out for three years. One college year was spent in London so I could flee the abject boredom of the Widener campus and hang out in English pubs. (Great cultural experience that British pub culture!) I learned a lot of wisdom sipping pints of Guinness Stout in these pubs.

During my academic matriculation at Widener I had two encounters that set me on my path to appreciating alternative healing. I'm telling you these stories not to bore you with my misspent youth, but to show you how a meat and potatoes person eventually embraced natural healing. I think most people think this health stuff is a crock; like me in my youth.

The first opinion-changing event on healthcare came during my freshman year at Widener when my girlfriend was rooming with a young woman whose father, Dr. Peter De Marco, was in the newspapers on a frequent basis for using experimental drugs on patients with chronic diseases.

My girlfriend needed a topic for a journalism course and decided to do an exposé on the injustice of the medical establishment towards Dr. De Marco. At the same time we had a philosophy professor, Sophocles M. Sophocles (yes, his real name), who was living on borrowed time by being treated with the doctor's experimental drug to treat severe arterial blockages. Her roommate's dad was accused of being a "quack" by the medical establishment for using unorthodox treatments on sick people.

As professor Sophocles often said to us, "I was surrendered to oblivion by my heart doctors. I was given a death sentence, six months to live. I had given up all hope until I met Dr. Peter De Marco. Peter has saved my life". He mentioned this in class numerous times.

At the time I was taking his philosophy class, the good professor had outlived his death sentence by six years through the use of this "miracle drug" Dr. De Marco was injecting into him called Procaine PVP.

This real life story of my professor using an experimental drug, bucking the medical establishment and surviving for many, many years past his predicted death, gave me a whole new perspective on alternative healing and so-called "quack" doctors. So did the medical establishment's aggressive persecution of Peter De Marco. My girlfriend and I arranged a visit to Dr. De Marco's office and clinic. It was an amazing, eye-opening experience for us. We were shown his laboratory where he had lab rats and mice in various states of disease being treated with injections of Procaine PVP. The diseased lab animals were all recovering from their ailments. He then took out a photo album with before and after photos of patients with gangrene. Incredible! Shocking photos of rotting, black, puss-filled, infected gangrenous limbs. Fingers, hands and feet rotting, were disintegrating painfully off of patients' bodies. These were some of the most grotesque photos I had ever seen. Then Dr. De Marco showed us photos taken weeks after injections of Procaine PVP were administered to these same patients. Miraculously, complete healing had occurred in all cases. There was complete repair of the infected, rotting tissue.

The limbs were healed and skin was regenerating. Dr. De Marco told us something that I was told was impossible: the body was regenerating cells. Taking damaged cells and building new, healthy cells. Miraculous! I have found a few natural remedies that do similar things. At this time in my life I thought "Once damaged and dying, cells are going to die."

We discussed the leading edge work that Dr. De Marco was performing on patients who were written off by their doctors while suffering tremendous pain, as well as the horror of watching their hands and legs rot away before their eyes.

The New Jersey State Medical Board dismissed Dr. De Marco's Procaine PVP therapy and worked to have his medical license revoked. The medical establishment's "not invented here" syndrome at work. This was my first witness to the tyranny and insanity of the medical establishment. Here you have helpless souls dying a slow, ugly, painful death being healed with an off-beat medicine while the medical establishment works to shut down the innovator who is saving lives of people who are in a desperate situation. "Why?" I asked. If your fingers, hand, arm, foot or leg are literally slowly, painfully disintegrating off your body, wouldn't you resort to anything to make it stop? Dr. De Marco was treating some of the most desperate patients who had run out of options and were obviously not getting relief from conventional therapy. Based on the time-phased photographs that I saw in his clinic, these poor souls were healing and getting better.

This was my first encounter with alternative medicine and the wrath that the medical establishment can reign in on healers who do not play by their rules. Dr. De Marco was labeled a dangerous quack by the authorities, in spite of overwhelming evidence that he was providing an invaluable service to his patients. They were getting relief.

My professor was living way past his predicted death date. I saw hundreds of files of clinical studies in Dr. De Marco's file cabinet. There were stacks of thank you letters from heart patients and gangrene sufferers testifying to their miraculous recoveries.

Granted, this was an experimental chemical compound, but my feeling is that you should be free to take whatever works to heal yourself and stop suffering. Take whatever resonates with your body. It's your life, not some bureaucrat's life.

"Freedom of choice." Isn't that what the United States Constitution, the greatest document created by man, says? So why are our freedoms being abridged?

Ironically, Procaine PVP is now widely accepted as a human growth hormone, as well as an anti-aging drug used by many people. Look it up on the Internet and you will see that this compound is now readily available to anyone. I don't know, what happened in the past 30 years? Someone is making money. In any case, this is the experience that got me to thinking. What else are we missing in medicine that we do not know about? Are there other healing secrets that are being kept away from us by the medical authorities? My suspicion was-yes there are.

The Refugee

The next brush with alternative healing came during my senior year at college. I was listening to Spanish tapes in the language lab that was located in the cellar of the college library. A below ground dungeon symbolically as well as in my own reality. There was an interesting Eastern European gentleman who ran the lab.

He was generally ignored by the majority of the students who considered him insignificant and custodian of the torture tapes. Nothing more tedious than listening to cassette tapes of conversational Spanish when you are an impatient, hot blooded college student.

Listening to foreign language tapes is as close to Chinese water torture as you can get for a college student, or anyone for that matter; very monotonous. There are pallets worth of my unlistened - to foreign language tapes in a landfill somewhere.

One day, out of a combination of boredom and curiosity, I approached the lab administrator and asked him his story. He was an elfish looking little fellow of about five feet five inches tall in stature, skinny, but with a handsome face accentuated by a thick, oversized handlebar mustache which was a source of great pride to him. The giant mustache was his signature look. He looked like the Keebler Elf. As far as I know, though, he never baked a chocolate chip cookie in his life.

He wore the same grey trousers and green plaid flannel shirt with a brown overcoat in all weather. It could be 80 degrees out and you'd see him striding across campus in his green plaid flannel shirt, overcoat and a golf cap on his head. He had a long extended stride, like the cartoon character "Mr. Natural". Very fitting! A wide extended, exaggerated gait. You've seen these people. They are over-dressed, no matter what the temperature or occasion. His name was Mikhail Miko.

Mikhail grew up during the Russian Revolution. So, counting back to the 1917 revolution, he was at least sixty years old when I met him in 1977. The stories he told me about the brutality of the revolution made my blood curdle.

As a young boy of ten years old, his father was instructed go to St. Petersburg (later Leningrad) from his village to witness disciplinary actions that would be taken against anyone who sympathized with the Bolshevik (communist) uprising. The White Russians, Czar Nicholas's people had a trench dug by accused Bolshevik sympathizer prisoners. He explained to me how they built a wooden platform at the edge of the trench and placed a butcher's table at the edge so that body parts could easily be tossed into the ditch below. Mikhail told me that he was forced to watch as men, women and children had ears, fingers, hands, arms and heads chopped off with a butcher's meat cleaver. The selected body part depended upon their suspected role or rank in the Bolshevik army or the offense that their family had allegedly perpetrated against the Czar's regime, or the whim of the torturer. Many innocent people were tortured as an example of what could happen to people who fought against the Czar.

Can you imagine being ten years old and witnessing this? Can you imagine taking your children to see this under threat of execution?

Following these atrocities, he witnessed equally brutal tortures from the other side; executions against the Czarists by the Bolsheviks against led by Joseph Stalin. In his youth, between 1916 and 1920, he was a witness to the lowest forms of human sufferings and depredations that were totally insane, arbitrary, traumatic, unbelievably taxing and sad. A living nightmare he never fully recovered from. These images ended the innocence of youth.

After the Bolsheviks conquered Russia, things settled down a little for Mikhail. He went to a university where he studied English and became a language teacher. The English lessons would later save his life and pave his way for resettlement in the U.S.

When World War II broke out, Mikhail was again subjected to starvation, violence and pain, this time at the hands of the Nazi German army during its attack on Russia. Mikhail, who was an English teacher at the time, was taken prisoner by the invading German army and shipped by rail car to Germany to work in a military ammunition factory with many other Russian civilians. He was manufacturing bombs and bullets that would be used against his own people back on the Russian front by Nazi soldiers. During his years in the Nazi factory prison he suffered from malnutrition, depression, dysentery, parasites and other illnesses that prisoners of war during World War II suffered at the hands of the Nazis.

After liberation, Mikhail was sent, by the Allies, to a displaced persons camp with many other refugees. He was going to be returned back to Russia. Mikhail had learned that Joseph Stalin, the Soviet Premier, had declared that many of the captured Russians on German soil were traitors, Nazi sympathizers, and, therefore, would be dealt with harshly(read: tortured, imprisoned, and murdered.), if they returned home.

Mikhail was spared, because he could speak German, Russian, and English. He talked his way into being an interpreter. He became useful to the Allied troops as a translator during the partition of Germany into East and West after World War II. He could facilitate discussions between the Russians, Americans, and Germans in his three languages.

Fortunately for Mikhail, his service to the Allies during the partition of Germany was recognized and he was rewarded with free passage to the United States. Returning to the Soviet Union was not an option, as surely he would have been imprisoned, tortured, and possibly put to death by Joseph Stalin's enforcers. Well-educated intellectuals, like Mikhail, were targeted for execution.

Mikhail gratefully accepted the passage to America, even though he yearned for his family in Russia.

When he arrived here in America, the effects of malnutrition, abuse, parasites, family separation, and forty years of struggle gave him severe bleeding stomach ulcers. Conventional doctors here in America attempted to treat him with allopathic medicine. His body did not respond and the condition worsened. Ultimately, the doctors wanted to remove a section of his stomach and fill him up with drugs. He almost died in the process.

In an act of desperation and last ditch attempt, Mikhail turned to alternative medicine. He found a Naturopath doctor (one of the few still around after Flexner) who diagnosed his condition and recommended a restricted vegetarian diet, combined with organic, raw, unpasteurized milk, golden seal powder, and myrrh powder. He told me that he took this for three months. The result, his stomach ulcers were completely healed and the parasites gone from his body.

Once his condition was healed, he continued the remedy once a week for the next thirty years. In addition to the herbs goldenseal, and myrrh, he took massive amounts of garlic (which you could smell coming through his pores and on his breath). Mikhail claimed that the herbs along with a vegetarian diet helped cure his sicknesses and, to some degree, helped with his emotional health.

Mikhail's story and life experience convinced me that there must be some merit to herbal remedies and natural, alternative healing. His return from a near-death condition to health, after conventional medicine failed him, struck a chord with me. It also taught me that no matter how bad you think your life situation is, there is always someone who is carrying a much heavier burden. Thank God for every small blessing that I have.

So the best lessons that I learned at Widener College had nothing at all to do with academics. They were: (1) you can cure sickness with nature, (2) a sense of gratitude that I never had before for being born in a peaceful time to a good family in America. His life story taught me a lot about healing and the human condition.

I started to take golden seal and myrrh (bad idea - as these are powerful, short duration herbs) just for the hell of it and started shopping at the local health food store for some of my groceries. My awareness of the potential benefits of natural healing was born.

"The Hippie"

The next flirtation with natural healing came in 1984 while I was employed in a high tech sales job working on a $33 million enterprise sales transaction. This was going to be the largest deal in the company's history and a "must win" opportunity to help slow the company's slide into oblivion. I was only twenty-seven years old at the time, with the weight of the world on my shoulders. My boss reminded me every day how important this deal was for the future of the company. My life, my career, my reputation depended on this deal closing – so I thought at the time.

In 1980 I started at Control Data Corporation, a well-respected $4 billion member of the Fortune 500, straight out of college. They were an innovator of computer-based education, online real estate listings, computer time sharing, data services, super computing, computer networking, mass storage systems, and owned a financial services company, Commercial Credit Corporation that Sandy Weil bought and built into CitiGroup. CDC spawned many successful companies that are still thriving today. Unfortunately, at the time that I joined the company, it was in a death spiral due to the predatory business practices of a giant competitor (guess who), as well as cronyism and mismanagement at corporate headquarters in Minneapolis, Minnesota. It was a great company, under a lot of pressure to survive. With this backdrop of financial pressure, deals like my big one got a lot of attention from executive management on "mahogany row." Weekly executive inquiries were coming down to me. This put a lot of pressure on me.

A combination of business stress, bad road food, late nights, partying, and too many airports left me with an ulcer that required medical treatment. I started out using over-the-counter antacids, then finally broke down and went to a doctor. The pain in my stomach was excruciating. I could not sleep or take my mind off the pain in my stomach.

I made an appointment with a general practitioner. The doctor gave me a prescription for an ulcer drug and referred me to a gastroenterologist (stomach doctor) who set me up for an upper GI (gastrointestinal) exam. You know, swallow dye, and then have X-rays to see what's going on. Mikhail's experience with his ulcer was ringing in my mind. The thought, however remote, of having part of my stomach removed, or any invasive procedure, was unsettling, even though his drastic circumstances were no match for my own.

I was taking golden seal and myrrh gum, according to Mikhail's remedy but couldn't find any raw, organic whole milk. It probably wouldn't have mattered because I was drinking a lot of beer at the time and had a lousy American diet. Nothing but a real change in lifestyle would really help me.

During my post-examination train ride home to the Philadelphia suburbs on the Paoli Local, I sat next to a hippie (aka long haired, counter culture, free-thinking guy). Good things happen to me on trains. I met my wife Linda on this same train, three years later.
He was probably under the influence or in possession of mind-altering products. I do recall that he was a very articulate and thoughtful person, with keen insights into natural healing.

The hippie and I got to talking. I told him about the pain that I was in and the dreaded upper GI that was scheduled in two weeks. He told me to skip the hospital and visit the Macrobiotic Center at the East West Foundation at 8th and South Streets in Philadelphia. He said that my ulcer was a manifestation of the way I way eating, thinking, and living. Through diet, meditation, and exercise I could cure anything. Macrobiotics was the answer, he assured me. The strange name "Macrobiotics" turned me off, but this thoughtful stranger got me thinking about alternative remedies for my ulcer.

The same week as the Hippie encounter, I ran into my brother's friend Geoff during a touch football game at Arnold Field in my boyhood town of Ardmore, Pa., the site of many important football and baseball games in my youth…and other youthful high jinks which I will not go into here.

Geoff was living a Macrobiotic lifestyle with his wife and dining at the East-West Foundation Center, the same place that the hippie and I had discussed. What a coincidence, I thought, to hear the word "Macrobiotics" two times in the same week, a term that I had never heard before. Now I know there is no such thing as "coincidence." Everything happens for a reason. This was a message from somewhere and I received it.

Geoff's wife was a high fashion model who regularly commuted between New York, Paris and Milan for photo shoots and shows. She needed to stay healthy and keep her weight down in order to remain in this highly competitive business. Some of her fellow fashion models were using drugs or going on starvation diets to maintain their tiny, skinny body shapes. His wife found macrobiotics a safe, healthy way to maintain her figure and avoid sickness from all of the international travel and jet-set abuse.

One night, while his wife was out of town, Geoff invited me to dinner and suggested that I try Macrobiotics out for a few weeks to see if it would work on curing my ulcer.

I made a beeline down to the East-West Foundation to see if I could postpone the uranium milk shake, x-rays, and chemical cocktails that were in store for me with the upper GI.

At that time, South Street was a very edgy, counter-culture Mecca where you could rub elbows with artists, musicians, poets, punk rockers, transvestites, bikers, panhandlers, jugglers, and all sorts of interesting characters. Today this area has been somewhat gentrified by the corporate chain stores, but still maintains some of its funky charm.

The East-West Foundation was on the second floor of an old building. The Foundation borrowed some of the character from the South Street scene below. (It was like the bar in the first Star Wars movie; kind of a freak show.) Businesswomen, hippies, sick people, cancer patients, palm readers, children, drug addicts, doctors, lawyers…all sorts of characters. There was this cult-like feel to the place. It was about the food, Laws of the Universe, and the consciousness that comes about as a result of following this diet. I wasn't ready for higher consciousness at that time – I just wanted a non-invasive way to cure my stomach ulcer so that I could get back to my partying ways. At this time I was a bachelor making decent money and spending it as fast as I could chasing women; mostly in bars and clubs around Philly. Not a great life or healthy lifestyle, but it was my life at the time; probably not that different from most young American males)

The food at the Foundation was very satisfying. The healing stories from the patrons about this diet were even better. They got me believing that my body could heal itself with the proper nutrition and attitude.

I bought and read *Macrobiotics,* by Michio Kushi, and took cooking lessons with a girl I was dating at the time. Believe me, I was very self-conscious taking cooking classes. I hid this cooking class business from my friends and family for years. This was a well kept secret, lest I expose my soft, feminine side. Me? Taking cooking classes? You've got to be kidding! Macrobiotic cooking lessons? My girlfriend actually thought it was a cool thing to do, so I scored some points doing something that I was otherwise embarrassed about.

Taking cooking classes was a severe challenge to my masculine side, but the pain in my stomach was so bad that I would have bought the entire Liza Minelli show tunes record collection, if I thought it would make me feel better. I would have bought and worn a Liberace gold lame jumpsuit…I would have placed a Freddy Mercury photo by my hearth…anything to get this ulcer monkey off my back. (Remember the movie Monkey on my Back? It's a classic. Rent it if you can find it. It must be watched after two in the morning in a semi-delirious state for full effect as I did in my misspent youth.)

The appointment with the gastroenterologist was cancelled. After speaking with a number of recovering cancer patients at the East-West Foundation, I was convinced that this diet was going to heal my sore stomach. Within three weeks of starting on the macrobiotic diet my ulcer was completely healed.

Once cured of my ulcer, I quit the macrobiotic diet and went back to drinking, partying, and carrying on. How quickly one forgets. I was a converted believer in natural healing based on this successful experience and followed it up with additional healing experiences that are shared in this book.

I never lost sight of the power of macrobiotics and incorporated some of the basic concepts into my life from that point forward.

Today, when I feel lousy, I go on a low acid, semi-macrobiotic diet until I feel better. I also eat locally grown, organic produce, and eat 75% vegetables and a modest amount of grains. I have made significant reductions in refined flour, sugars, processed foods, and cut way back on the use of pharmaceuticals. So I did make a few lifestyle changes after my initial macrobiotic experience. I became infinitely more aware of my diet, combined with being conscious of my thought patterns and their impact on my health.

I was on to something, but was not ready to completely reform myself.

In the midst of succumbing to the ulcer due to corporate stress, in addition to the macrobiotic diet, I learned how to meditate and blow off steam with physical exercise. The adrenalin and cortisol that your glands are spewing into your system from stress will poison you. I found a few healthy ways to blow off steam (besides drinking alcohol) to reduce stress. Stress is by far the greatest cause of sickness in our society today. Find healthy ways to blow off built-up stress.

One more recent story

"Your cholesterol is high…Here, take these pills for the rest of your life"

In 2005, I had a complete physical, including stress test and blood work. The stress test indicated that I had the cardiovascular strength of the average male in his 20s. This was gratifying. The technicians at the stress test lab questioned why I was even recommended for the test since it was not reimbursed by medical insurance unless you had a chronic condition. I had been told that, since I have a family history of heart problems, that I should retain a cardiologist to monitor my mid-life cardiac health and that a stress test would be covered since I was an "at-risk" patient. I ended up with $500 in uncovered medical expense for the stress test, but gained some peace of mind knowing that my heart was in decent shape.

The surprise on the downside of this physical exam was that my cholesterol was a whopping 260! Very high! I had no idea it was that high. A reading this high is considered to be in the danger zone. Statistically you have a higher chance of a heart attack or a stroke the higher the number gets past 220.

My physician advised that I was in the "high risk" category for a heart attack and needed to begin taking statin drugs. A prescription for Lipitor™ was given to me. Statin drugs are now some of the most widely prescribed drugs in the United States and are effective in lowering LDL (bad) cholesterol. But, I asked myself, is the cure worse than the ailment? I know, Dr. Jarvick, the genius who invented the artificial heart, uses statin drugs as do many others. This guy Dr. Jarvick may be a genius, but I'm personally not buying into this drug thing. It's my personal choice. Do you believe everything you hear on TV? I don't.

Statin drugs work by blocking the enzyme that your liver needs to produce LDL. They do not have much of an effect on HDL or good cholesterol. Pravachol, Zocor, and Mevacor are also statin drugs that are prescribed by doctors to lower cholesterol or to prevent high cholesterol in "high risk" patients like me.

What do you think I did? Run to the pharmacy like 80% of "high risk," fearful patients do when a doctor tells them they need a drug with some harmful side effects? Of course not! I threw the prescription in the trash can on the way out of the doctor's office, and then set out to clear my arteries. I do not recommend that you follow my lead on this unless you consult with a naturopath and get on a prescribed cholesterol regime.

I researched statin drugs and discovered that they have serious side effects in some people, including causing liver damage. Other potential side effects are muscle pains, headaches, and impotence. "Sorry Doc, this ain't for me." I'm pretty sure that a lot of lives have been saved by the use of statin drugs, just not mine. Not right now, maybe someday?

There are a lot of natural compounds in food and supplements that can help lower cholesterol naturally in people. The challenge with all this stuff is that you need to find out what works for you. In my case, the cholesterol is both hereditary and lifestyle/diet-related. I can do something about the second factor, but very little about the first.

Right around the time I had the physical, I discovered colonics and Dr. Bernard Jensen's writings on health. One of his main premises (which I now believe) is all disease starts in the digestive tract and colon. I went on a massive cleansing effort and fast to rid my body of 40+ years of toxins. Toxins end up in your blood stream, affecting all of your systems, including your arteries and heart. I reasoned that I could shave a few points of cholesterol off my high count just by getting "clean". Another part of this colon care deal was consuming high-fiber foods like flaxseed, oatmeal, and brown rice. They act as a sponge and draw some of the fats out of your system.

The other thing that I began religiously was to take Omega 3 fish oils. For fiber I primarily use whole or milled flaxseeds, which are both high in fiber and Omega 3 and 6 fatty acids. Omega 3 helps increase the level of HDL cholesterol and decrease LDL.

Garlic (active ingredient, allicin), green tea, and healthy oils, like olive and grape seed, became the exclusive cooking oils in our home. We will occasionally use sesame seed oil and walnut oil.
I never liked deep fried food, so the dreaded hydrogenated oils were never something I needed to worry about.

For me, red meat consumption, which has not been really high for twenty years, went down to two meals per week. When consumed it is lean, grass-fed meat only. I make an exception on certain road trips when I'm at a steakhouse, but this is pretty rare. I eat chicken and fish two times per week and mostly vegetables the rest of the time, following a combination blood type/macrobiotic diet. Recently, I drastically cut carbs in my diet reducing my glycemic resistance, which also contributes to cardiovascular health.

I eat dairy in the form of grass-fed goat cheese and eat regular cow's milk cheese only occasionally.

My exercise regime, a minimum of three days per week of moderate to vigorous cardio and weight training, has been continuously followed for twenty years. Exercise is key.

So, without any drugs, I successfully lowered my cholesterol 24 points in one year.. If I were more disciplined, and really cut out all fatty food, coffee, alcohol, and occasional binge eating, I believe my cholesterol would be another 20 points lower, in the 210 range, which is ideal for me. You can't stop enjoying life, but I plan on finding a healthy short cut to getting there.

My new cholesterol target is 210 - and I will achieve this with minimal dietary changes. I plan to try some natural, cholesterol lowering supplements that my naturopathic doctor has prescribed.
So the lesson in this story is, there are alternatives to prescription drugs, in some cases. For me, finding a natural alternative to prescription drugs is the best path. Consult your physician about alternatives that may work for you.

These accounts are not meant to be taken as medical advice. These are my own personal stories that I am sharing as learning experiences for the reader and insights into how a conventional medicine-focused person found solutions in alternative medicine. Consult your physician or health provider in all medical matters. The use of prescription drugs may be necessary for certain conditions. I don't make any medical recommendations in this book, as I am not a trained physician.

Chapter 21
Your Present Medical Beliefs and How They Got There: The Flexner Report

"Although there is no progress without change, not all change is progress."
— John Wooden

Here's the revealing story of how a high school principal changed our healthcare system and the way you are treated today in the United States of America and Canada and anywhere in the world that Allopathic medicine is practiced.

Did you ever wonder how our present-day American medical establishment got started? Why you are treated the way you are and the consequences of this way of healing?

Here's the short story. Not many people know this story so check it out. As you start reading this, think about everything you've ever been told about your health and medicine. It's incredible to me that one man and one report on medicine changed our lives the way this one has. First, a few questions for you:

- Why do drug companies want to force neutraceutical manufacturers and vitamin manufacturers into requiring a prescription? Read here about the Codex Alimentarius regulations that are coming if we don't get off our keisters and fight.

- Why do the American Medical Association (AMA) and Federal Drug (FDA) fight so hard to keep natural cures out of the hands of ordinary people?

- Why is nutrition a neglected short course in most medical school curricula? It is no accident most hospital food looks and tastes like airline food. And these are healing establishments? With this excuse for food?

- How come Chiropractors, Homeopaths, Naturopaths, and Osteopaths were scorned by the medical establishment and sent underground in the early 1900s? What is allopathic medicine and why should we care?

Allopathic Medicine, also known as "conventional medicine," is the medical approach which seeks to cure by producing a condition in the body different than, or opposite to, the condition that exists within the diseased state. It is the most common method in the United States. It is also the one taught in most medical schools and practiced by the medical doctors (MDs) America. There is a high reliance on pharmaceutical drugs and surgery to correct illness.

Naturopathic Medicine is a practice that seeks to use the body's natural capabilities to heal itself with a variety of treatments, including nutrition, herbs, natural foods, acupuncture, hydrotherapy, homeopathy, light therapy, and other natural remedies. It is the primary focus of this book and my personal preferred method of healing.

Homeopathic Medicine is a branch of naturopathic medicine that relies on three basic principles: (1) like cures like, (2) minimal dose, and (3) a single remedy is used.

Why have people become brainwashed that prescription drugs and costly, sometimes unnecessary, surgery are the only way to cure illness and get better? Do you think all of this is an accident?

I, like some of you, are baffled by the contradictions and ignorance that permeates the practice of medicine in the United States. Things are slowly getting better, but not fast enough for me. Allopathic medicine is the best at these eight things, in my opinion:

Allopathic Medicine at its Best

1. Emergency and Critical Care
2. Diagnostic technology: Blood tests, X-rays, Ultrasound, and CAT scans
3. Orthopedics: Joint replacement and arthroscopic surgery
4. Pain Management
5. Surgery: Cosmetic and Corrective
6. Pediatrics: Infant care and corrective surgery
7. Biotechnology, as it relates to curing genetic diseases

Where allopathic medicine falls short is in the areas of nutrition, preventative medicine, over-use of pharmaceuticals, unnecessary surgeries, and, in many cases, a complete ignorance of natural healing modalities.

Allopathic Medicine Shortcomings

1. Heavy reliance and over-use of pharmaceutical drugs. Drug company incentives to doctors to prescribe drugs.
2. Unnecessary surgeries: Revenue generation for the practice
3. Botched surgeries: Careless mistakes in the operating room
4. Mis-diagnosis of ailments leading to worse suffering; prescribing one drug after another, hoping something eventually

works before poisoning the patient with chemicals.

5. Targeting symptoms instead of looking at the whole person; not looking at the whole mind, body, and spiritual condition of the patient

6. Bacterial mutations: Antibiotic-resistant strains of bacteria that have evolved as a result of over-prescribing antibiotics to patients. Certain hospitals are now breeding grounds for these virilant strains of bacteria. You introduce health risk by entering a hospital where you are supposed to be healing yourself; 80,000 Americans die each year as a result of infectionsacquired while in the hospital. (Trust me. It's better to stay out of the hospital, if you can.)

How did the medical system get this way in the United States? Where do our beliefs on healing and health come from? I could never figure this out until I stumbled upon an old report and then it all came together for me. **The Flexner Report:** Our American Collective Consciousness of Allopathic Medicine[1] This is a short story on how your medical system got to be what it is today.

So how did we get to our present 21st Century beliefs about medicine and healing? Part of the answer is the Flexner Report and the institutions that used the report to support massive changes in the United States and Canadian medical establishment. Never heard of it? Well neither did I until I stumbled upon it in the course of my research.

A Short Historical Perspective

Back in the good old days, which really were not very good from a healthcare vantage point, there was a proliferation of different medical practices in America. Some of it was good, most of it was

---

1 Flexner, Abraham, *Medical Education in the United States and Canada,* New York, NY Carnegie Foundation, 1910.

bad. The practice of "bleeding" a patient until she gets better (or dies) is probably the worst old - time remedy that I'm happy is gone. Not all of the treatments were this whacky, but there was plenty of room for improvement.

There was also an unregulated patent medicine industry that, in some cases, was selling toxic remedies which sometimes killed consumers. Anyone with some glass bottles, alcohol, and other ingredients could sell a remedy to an uneducated public.

In the mid 1800s there was no sterilization, sanitation, or knowledge of germs.

The American Civil War (1861–1865), for the first time, shed light on the need for sterilization and sanitation in the United States. Diseases were the biggest killers during the Civil War, not bullet wounds. Army surgeons did not know how to sterilize medical instruments, so disease and infection were readily transferred from physician to patient and patient-to-patient through dirty hands, bandages, and unsterile instruments.

Sewage and garbage were dumped within close proximity to army camps which created a breeding ground for a number of diseases. This lack of cleanliness was gradually recognized as the root cause. Sickness spread through army camps like wildfire.

In 1867, Joseph Lister identified airborne bacteria as a cause of disease and used carbolic spray for surgical sterilization. It was also around this time that sewage systems were being built in major towns and cities in the United States.

Medical schools in the late 1800s had very lax admission standards and no standard curriculum. Most of the physicians were trained as apprentices, for varying amounts of time. They had no clinical or laboratory experience and textbooks were few and far between. Everyone was teaching medical students in a different manner. The use of basic diagnostic tools, like stethoscopes and microscopes, was rare as were standard procedures for treating disease.

Hospitals in those days were crowded and were no more sanitary than the Civil War Field Hospitals. They were breeding grounds for disease and were to be avoided at all costs.

So given this set of conditions, a massive change was needed to upgrade and improve all aspects of medicine. Abraham Flexner, a high school principal, was hired by the Carnegie Foundation to research medical practices and published a report with the backing of the newly formed American Medical Association (AMA). The recommendations in his report were taken and served as the catalyst for major changes in medicine that are still in effect today. The changes suggested by Flexner in some cases were positive, such as:

- Using the scientific method to research, diagnose, and treat disease so that there was a standard, repeatable process.

- Understanding and acceptance of germ theory. Acceptance that germs and their spread causes many diseases. Using microscopes and laboratories to research and formulate new, innovative pharmaceutical medicines.

- The need for sanitation and sterilization to reduce the growth and spread of contagious disease in hospitals.

- Higher academic standards for admission into medical schools.

- Standard curriculum for all medical schools. This was both good and bad for the practice of medicine.

- Closure of sub-standard hospitals and medical schools.

The Flexner Report also helped create the pharmaceutical industry as we know it today. It gave the AMA tremendous power and influence. In addition, Flexner helped give birth to the Food and Drug Administration (FDA). These are the foundation of today's American medical establishment. So for better and worse our medical system was changed in the early 20th century.

Both of these organizations were created with the goal of improving medical practices, protecting the public interest, and improving society. In many ways they succeeded in this mission. Where they failed (like many well-intentioned governmental programs) was in the sweeping changes that they enforced in multiple areas. Here is a partial list:

- Flexner sanctioned allopathic medicine as the only legitimate school of medicine. Allopathic medicine is the practice of treating disease with remedies which produce effects different from those under treatment. Use the opposite remedy to cure the disease and treat symptoms rather than the whole person. MDs' use allopathic or "conventional medicine" regimens to treat their patients. This is probably 90% of the doctors in the United States.

- Flexner repudiated homeopathic medicine which treats disease with remedies (in minute doses) to create the same symptoms as the disease being treated. It is natural and very effective for most patients.

- Flexner also stigmatized Osteopathy, Chiropractic, and Eastern medicine.

- The advocacy of pharmaceutical-based remedies, with very little credence given to diet, nutrition, herbs, energy medicine, and faith healing.

- Treating the symptoms of disease rather than healing the whole person, ignoring, in many cases, the root cause of the disease. Throwing drugs at a problem instead of dealing with underlying emotional or spiritual aspects of the individual.

- Heavy emphasis on surgical procedures when a natural remedy could potentially save an organ and the trauma associated with invasive surgery.

- Increased the cost structure of healthcare by raising tuition in medical schools, while closing down others, thereby impacting the supply and demand equation, such that costs on every level increased for medical treatment.

- The formation of an unholy alliance of the AMA, FDA, medical schools, and pharmaceutical industry that does not always have the public's best interests at heart and persecutes alternative healers for breaking with allopathic medical practices.

- License to a total revamp of medical schools, text books, education, hospitals, budgets, and, most importantly, pushing natural medicine underground.

The curse of medical knowledge and the birth of bought and paid for medicine, starts here.

The curse of knowledge refers to the human tendency to assimilate a set of beliefs that become ingrained in the mind and then block all new ideas and patterns of thinking that are contrary to one's present knowledge. This is what happened with Flexner. It became fixed in our minds and now it is very difficult for most people to accept new, better ways of thinking about healing. Our minds have "calcified" or frozen into believing allopathic medicine is the only right way of healing. This same curse of knowledge exists in religion, politics, ethnicity, nationalism, and many other human endeavors to our collective detriment. It's the "Well, that's the way it's always been done" dead-end trap.

The Flexner Report, though well intentioned, eliminated many branches of the healing arts from our health system with extremely bad consequences. There are quacks and phonies in every realm of human activity. They exist in allopathic and naturopathic medicine as well, so I'm not implying that there is a perfect answer anywhere.

Rather than selectively weeding out the quacks, substandard hospitals, and medical schools, the AMA and medical establishment mowed the entire field down to the dirt. Using Flexner as a roadmap, they replaced a collection of good healing practices with one: allopathic medicine. As a result, you have limited choices in the kind of treatment you can receive and a limited set of choices that health insurance providers will cover.

I have spent over $20,000 out-of-pocket on Reiki, acupuncture, herbs, PC therapy, nutrition, radiances, colon hydrotherapy, nutritional counseling and other natural healing modes because my medical insurance does not recognize alternative healing. By doing these responsible things I am saving the system thousands of dollars in present and future medical expenses. If I had submitted healthcare claims for thousands of dollars of pharmaceuticals they would have happily paid my claim. I believe, in spite of the naturopathic treatment expenses, this is money well invested. The healthcare system we have has to change. It is totally out of whack.

The Flexner Report opened the avenue for corporate greed to manipulate the rules of the game to their advantage and profits. This is called "bought and paid for science." This is how a pharmaceutical company can get a drug approved for public consumption by the FDA even when there is a long laundry list of known life-threatening side effects, including some that can kill you. Just look at the drug advertisements on television and listen to the talking heads explain the multiple side effects that some of these approved drugs can cause.

Go to the Internet and look up the news on Zeta. The news you will read about the lawsuits against the drug companies will confirm what I'm saying here.

Colon hydrotherapy, Reiki, and all manner of energy healing techniques are strictly regulated by the government and are not reimbursed by medical insurance even though they are proven to heal people.

The pharmaceutical industry, FDA, and AMA have conspired to keep alternative healing methods underground for years because of the profits that would be lost if people would look after themselves better and had access to nature's healing bounty. I made a conscious decision to spend my own money to heal myself rather than rely on a system that is broken and corrupt in many areas. The pharmaceutical drugs prescribed to me during several illnesses were harming me as much as the illnesses did.

I continue to use allopathic medicine, as does my family, but use it sparingly and only after all natural avenues have been explored. There are many more good things than bad things in conventional medicine so I don't want to leave the impression that I am against it. Big business and government regulations are the two things that have corrupted an otherwise noble institution. I will add the insurance industry and legal profession as two other groups who are part of the problem with healthcare.

Supporting evidence for what I am saying about a conspiracy to control natural medicine can be found in the campaign to pass the Codex Alimentarius.

Codex Alimentarius: Restricting your access to natural healing products[2]

Codex Alimentarius (Codex) was created in 1962 by the United Nations to control the international trade in food. It has morphed into a vehicle to regulate vitamins and supplements and potentially deprive consumers' access to these products. The Codex regulations are enforced by the World Trade Organization (WTO), which can impose sanctions on any country that does not comply. So, if Codex

---

2 Natural Solutions Foundation, www.healthfreedomus.org

goes into law on December 31, 2009, the WTO can levy hefty fines on the United States if we're still buying vitamins and supplements freely. Codex has written a set of guidelines that decreases the allowable dosages in vitamins and minerals to "reduce their toxicity" and their nutritional value. If you want an effective dose of vitamins and supplements, you will need a prescription.

Big pharma and chemical companies want to "protect" consumers from abusing nutritional supplements through the Vitamin and Mineral Guideline, which would significantly reduce the dosage and potency of nutritional products. Nutrients are considered dangerous toxins by Codex and therefore they should be controlled.

Codex is the sickness industry's attempt to cut off natural healing alternatives to consumers so that you are forced to consume pharmaceuticals and other chemical-based medicines. Under Codex, your access to natural healing products will be severely limited. The duck blind that these "consumer advocates" are hiding in is the Council for Responsible Nutrition (CRN). This organization includes people from the pharmaceutical and chemical industries who are working tirelessly to slip the Codex rules into place by 2010 globally. If this happens, your free and easy access to vitamins and supplements will be curtailed.

The United States Congress passed the Dietary Supplement Health and Education Act (DSHEA) in 1994 that classifies supplements and herbs as food, which can not have an upper limit set on their use. This bill was passed by unanimous Congressional consent based on a massive drive by voters. If passed, Codex will over-ride the DSHEA. A bunch of foreign and domestic bureaucrats are trying to dictate to us what we can take. This is crazy, but it's real.

The Natural Solutions Foundation is lobbying to prevent Codex Alimentarius from being enacted. Take a few minutes. Check out the Natural Solution Foundation and support the cause of freedom of choice. Now who would deny you your personal rights to choose your own nutritional supplements? You know the answer.

More evidence of abuses by the "sickness" industry is documented in Gary Null's documentary, Prescription for Disaster, which is an in-depth investigation into the cooperation between the pharmaceutical industry, hospitals, and medical colleges. It exposes the inter-twined relationship between our health care providers and industry, that is having disastrous consequences on our health and the healthcare industry. Gary Null also authored Death by Medicine. He is an authority on the subject of conventional medicine practices and can provide you with detailed, fact-based evidence so you can draw your own conclusions, separate from the opinions of this author.

Another contributing factor to the problems in healthcare is the practice of defensive medicine by doctors who are afraid of malpractice lawsuits. Tort lawyers have created massive problems for doctors by filing frivolous lawsuits. Most lawsuits are totally unwarranted and are purely based on generating profits, not protecting wronged patients. Tort reform needs to be enacted so that doctors can get back to practicing medicine instead of constantly looking over their backs to see if an over zealous lawyer is preparing to sue them. Get out and vote for tort reform every chance you get. The ambulance-chasing lawyers have gotten out of hand. This has a huge negative impact on the way allopathic medicine is practiced today (all healing), since a doctor has to practice defensive medicine when treating you to protect himself.

The reason I include this chapter in my book is that many of you rely solely on the conventional medical industry for 100% of your care, like I did for many years. Some of you will not believe many things that I say in this book because your frame of reference was shaped (unknowingly) by decades of compliance to a dusty old report that Flexner published back in the early 1900s. So, now that you see how our collective consciousness has been molded by the legacy of the Flexner Report for 100 years, you are a free thinker, you will change some of your thoughts on medicine to your ultimate benefit.

To conclude: Healing is accomplished by whatever means the

patient requires or whatever resonates with his/her condition. No single method of healing, be it allopathic, naturopathic, homeopathic or any other modality holds the magic key. But you do need to make conscious, informed choices and know why the present system works the way it does.

Consider all options. Take control of your health and make choices based on what is best for you.

Helplessness is our Enemy

The obvious, but not so obvious, health fact ...

The pharmaceutical industry lays claim to having helped address most of the major diseases in the world. This is only partially true. In actual fact, the major breakthroughs in modern healthcare are the use of: sterilization processes, sewage treatment and disposal process, and water treatment systems. The World Health Organization has established that 80% of the diseases in the world are caused by unclean drinking water and, by extension, sewage disposal and treatment.

Historically, a large majority of human epidemics were a result of a lack of cleanliness in these areas, which we take for granted today in modern, industrialized countries.

Unclean water remains a massive disease problem today in third world countries. People often think our higher standard of health is due to huge medical technological breakthroughs that curbed diseases. It is and it isn't.

Cleaning up water supplies, washing hands, and disposing of refuse properly will generate 80% of the health benefit to people who are not eating the American fast food diet. It's not drugs that make you healthy; it's your water and healthy food. Fix these two things and you've nailed most of the health problems. The sources of the other 20%, in my opinion, are stress, environmental pollution, and genetic.

Why did man take 5,000 years to figure this out? Good health is actually pretty simple, if you live in a place that has clean water and access to natural food.

Point Counter Point

So my readers, do not think I am a shill for the naturopathy, I am going to provide a dissenting opinion. This is, of course, in the interests of fair and balanced reporting. Here is a contrary viewpoint regarding Homeopathy.

John Stossel's book *Myths, Lies, and Downright Stupidity* exposes many commonly held myths.[1] He tells a story about a millionaire who offered a cash reward of $1 million dollars to anyone who could prove conclusively that homeopathic medicine actually cures people. He says that the reward went unclaimed. Stossel also says that the highly popular homeopathic allergy and flu remedies flying off of shelves in pharmacies today have absolutely no healing value. To quote:

Myth: Homeopathy is a good treatment for allergies and the flu. Truth: Homeopathy is absurd.

Sadly, Americans are already kissing many millions good-bye. Every year, companies sell hundreds of millions of dollars worth of homeopathic remedies.

You know what? John Stossel is right. For some people homeopathy does not work for healing. For some people pharmaceuticals don't work. Contradictions in healing are common. Find what resonates with you. We're all right and we're all wrong.

Some other interesting things that Stossel covered in his book: Astrology: Stossel had an astrological chart done for Ed Kemper,

---

1 John Stossel, *Myths, Lies and Downright Stupidity*, New York, NY: Hyperion 2006 p213

Your Present Medical Beliefs and How They Got There: The Flexner Report   238

the convicted California serial killer and necrophile (one who has sex with corpses).[2] This miscreant Kemper murdered six female hitchhikers and his own mother. There is a point to this story, I promise.

Stossel gave Kemper's twenty-five page astrological report to a class of college students. The students were impressed and amazed at the accuracy of the report (Kemper's) as it applied to their own lives. "That's exactly me," some of the astonished students exclaimed after reading the astrological chart. Some of the students became believers in astrology based on these charts until Kemper's identity for the charts was revealed to them. This just goes to show how gullible the consuming public is. Like me, read the label before you buy; on everything. Don't be somebody's stooge. We're all stooges at one time or another. We just need to minimize our stoogery; in everything.

Personally, I believe there are benefits to astrology, but you have so much free will to change your life that astrology is just a nice very high-level guidance system; not a tool to rule your life. It's one more tool in the tool box, but not something to get nutty about. Some people get stupid with astrology. It's just another data point to be mixed with all the other data points in your life and should be weighed appropriately, in my opinion. It's pepper in your soup, not the broth or the key ingredient, just a spice.

Like everything in this life, medicine, religion, science, and politics, you are going to discover contradictions. Welcome to the real world. In this world there are only possibilities and probabilities, nothing is fixed or certain.

So I provide this information to show that you'll find contradictions everywhere in healing, just like in life.

---

2   John Stossel, *Myths, Lies and Downright Stupidity*, New York, NY: Hyperion 2006 Pages 206–207

Wrap Up
Roswell, New Mexico, April 15, 2008

I just walked into my hotel room on Main Street in Roswell, famous for the alien space craft that crashed in a field at a local ranch in an area known as the Plains of Augustin in early July, 1947.

I turned on the TV in my room at Danny's Dew Drop Inn and the Philadelphia Phillies beat the Houston Astros in the 9th inning. I pinch myself. Is all this happening? Is this real? Space aliens, a Phillies 9th inning come-from-behind win, and this book finally finished? I must be dreaming! The final touches to this book were made in Roswell, New Mexico which I find totally in keeping with the outer space undercurrents in some sections of *Rich Remedies, Volume 1*.

I hope that you enjoyed reading this book and learned a few things that are practical and that you can put to use to make your own life happier and healthier. If you have, then I have succeeded. My objective was to show you how I, with no background in natural healing, found solutions to some very pressing health problems by finding good healing coaches and doing my own independent research.

A second point that I hope you noticed is that I took control of my own situation and found healing solutions to some pretty annoying and at times debilitating sicknesses that I had. In this process I had to go against the grain of some standard procedures and buck the system to get well.

The final point that I hope you came to understand and will incorporate into your own life is the conscious use of energy in its many forms: thoughts, light, color, nutrition, bio-energetics, or any of the others discussed in this book. As energetic beings, we transmit and receive energy on a continual basis. Figure out what resonates with you and use this energy for your benefit.

I hope that you are able to take away some humor as well as learning from this book. I chuckle sometimes when I see myself swimming in the "deep end" of the alternative healing world. There are a lot of good, useful things to be learned as long as we maintain our perspective and at times a sense of humor, Thanks and as Paul Harvey says:

"And that's the rest of the story ... good day!"[1]

Thank You!

---

[1] *Paul Harvey is a syndicated radio host and author.*

Bibliography

Arntz, William, Betsy Chasse, and Mark Vincente. What the Bleep Do We Know!?: Discovering the endless possibilities for altering your everyday reality. Deerfield Beach, Fla: Health Communications, Inc., 2005.

Bioptron AG, Editors, Colour Therapy Basics, Switzerland

Breiling, Brian et al. Light Years Ahead. Berkeley,Ca:Light Years Ahead Publishing. 1996.

Center for Immune Research, Clinical Abstracts, httep://www. naturalinterferon. com/clinical html pages 1–4. All references to the clinical tests for NutriFeron® are provided by the CIR.

Cooper, Primrose. The Healing Power of Light. York Beach, ME: Weiser Books, Inc., 2001.

D'Adamo, Peter J., and Catherine Whitney. Eating Right 4 Your Type. New York: G.P. Putnam's Sons, 1996.

Dispenza, Joseph. Live Better Longer: The Parcells Center 7-Step Plan for Health and Longevity. Lincoln, Nebr: iUniverse.com, Inc. 2000

Duke, James A. PhD, *The Green Pharmacy Herbal Handbook.* New York, NY: Rodale Press 1997.

Emoto, Masaru. *The Hidden Messages in Water.* Hillsboro, Ore.: Beyond Words Publishing, Inc., 2004. Emoto, Masaru. *The Secret Life of Water.* Hillsboro, Ore.: Beyond Words Publishing, Inc., 2003.

Ferre, Carl, *Pocket Guide to Macrobiotics,* Berkley, Ca: Crossing Press, 1997.

Gienger, Michael. *Crystal Power, Crystal Healing.* New York: Sterling Publishing Co., 1998.

Haverford Wellness Center. website www.haverfordwellness.com/about

Grace, Meridian, N.D. *Awakening Health,* Austin, Texas. AwakeningHealth.com

Higa, Teruo, PhD. *Our Future Reborn.* Tokyo, Japan: Sunmark Publishing. 2006.

Jensen, Bernard. *Dr. Jensen's Guide to Better Bowel Care.* New York: Avery, Penguin Putman, 1999.

Kast, Terry, *Parcells Method of Healing,* P.O. Box 50010, Albuquerque, NM 87181

Kushi, Mishio, and Alex Jack. *The Book of Macro-Biotics.* Tokyo: Japan Publications, 1986.

Kushi, Mishio, and MarcVan Cauwenberghe. *Natural Healing Through Macrobiotics*. Japan: Japan Publications, 1978.Liberman, Jacob. *Light Medicine of the Future*. Rochester, Vt.: Bear & Company, 1991.

McGarey, William A.. *The Oil That Heals: A Physician's Successes with Castor Oil Treatments*. Virginia Beach: A.R.E. Press, 1993.

Newton, Michael. *Journey of Souls: Case Studies of Life Between Lives*. St. Paul, Minn.: Llewellyn Publications, 1994.

Siegel, Bernie, MD, *Love, Medicine & Miracles:*New York, NY.Harper & Row Publishers, 1986

Shaklee Corporation, NutriFeron® See www.shaklee.com/rich, NutriFeron®

Shealy, Norman,. and Dawson Church. *Soul Medicine: Awakening Your Inner Blueprint for Abundant Health and Energy*. Santa Rosa, Cal.: Elite Books, 2006.

Sugrue, Thomas. *There is a River: The Story of Edgar Cayce*. Virginia Beach: A.R.E.

Press, 1945.Teppone, Mikhail, M.D. AcuTech, International, Inc. info@acutechinternational.com.

Two Feather, William. *Medicine Man, Teacher, Healer, Musician, and Author*. http://www.2feather.com/home.html

Underwood, Anne, and Jerry Adler. "It isn't just what you eat that can Kill You, and it Isn't Just your DNA That Can Save You-It's How They Interact." *Newsweek*, January 24, 2005.

Waterworks4U.com, Dr. J. Belot PhD., Benefits ofr Ionized Water.

Weiss, Brian L., "Many Lives, Many Masters".New York, NY: Simon and Shuster.1988.

Weiss, Brian L. Same Soul, Many Bodies.New York, NY: Simon and Shuster,2004.

Yechiel E, Barenholzy.,J.Biol Chem 1985 Aug 5, 260 (16) :9123. Haverford Wellness Center, BodyBio Bulletin, part number 902.2, www.bodybio.com

Young, Robert, and Shelly Redford Young. The pH Miracle. New York: Warner Books, 2002.

Website and Resources:
www.richremedies.com

This is my website where I offer links to books, nutritional supplements, EM Technology™ solutions, water alkalizers, environmentally-friendly products healing merchandise, healing stories, my affiliates, and many other helpful resources.

About the Author

I have consciously researched and used natural healing remedies to cure myself from a variety of illnesses. I am sharing my experiences with those who may benefit from my years of experience and success. I live in Austin, Texas. Married with three children employed in high technology sales for 20 years.